The Business of Veterinary Practice

Edited by

JOHN SHERIDAN
Anicare Group Services, West Sussex

and

OWEN McCAFFERTY
North Olmstead, Ohio

PERGAMON PRESS

OXFORD · NEW YORK · SEOUL · TOKYO

U.K.	Pergamon Press Ltd., Headington Hill Hall, Oxford OX3 0BW, England
U.S.A.	Pergamon Press, Inc., 660 White Plains Road, Tarrytown, New York 10591-5153, U.S.A.
KOREA	Pergamon Press Korea, K.P.O. Box 315, Seoul 110-603, Korea
JAPAN	Pergamon Press Japan, Tsunashima Building Annex, 3-20-12 Yushima, Bunkyo-ku, Tokyo 113, Japan

First edition 1993

Library of Congress Cataloging-in-Publication Data
The Business of veterinary practice / edited by John Sheridan
and Owen McCafferty. – 1st ed.
p. cm. – (Pergamon veterinary handbook series)
1. Veterinary medicine–Practice. I. Sheridan, John.
II. McCafferty, Owen. III. Series.
SF756.4.B87 1993
636.089'068—dc20 92–41236

British Library Cataloguing in Publication Data
A catalogue record for this book is available
from the British Library.

ISBN 0-08-040846 X

DISCLAIMER

Whilst every effort is made by the Publishers to see that no inaccurate or misleading data, opinion or statement appear in this book, they wish to make it clear that the data and opinions appearing in the articles herein are the sole responsibility of the contributor concerned. Accordingly, the Publishers and their employees, officers and agents accept no responsibility or liability whatsoever for the consequences of any such inaccurate or misleading data, opinion or statement.

(M)636.089 068 S

Printed in Great Britain by B.P.C.C. Wheatons Ltd, Exeter.

The Business of Veterinary Practice

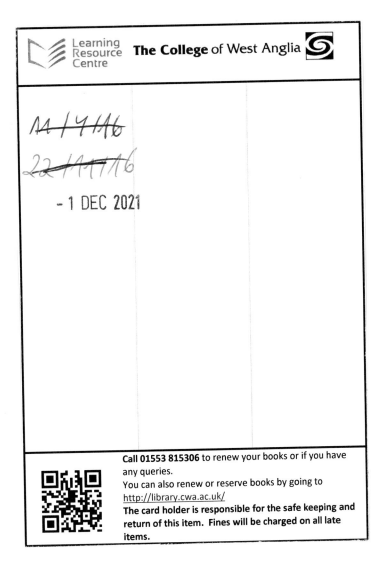

Learning Resource Centre — The College of West Anglia

11/4/16

22/11/16

- 1 DEC 2021

Call 01553 815306 to renew your books or if you have any queries.
You can also renew or reserve books by going to
http://library.cwa.ac.uk/
The card holder is responsible for the safe keeping and return of this item. Fines will be charged on all late items.

Pergamon Veterinary Handbook Series

Series Editor: A. T. B. Edney

This new series of practical and authoritative handbooks covers topics of interest to the practising veterinary surgeon, to veterinary students and to veterinary nurses. The text is authoritative, yet written in a clear and accessible form, and there are numerous photographs and specially commissioned line drawings to enhance understanding. The volumes in this series will be valuable additions to any practice bookshelf.

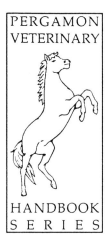

PERGAMON
VETERINARY

HANDBOOK
SERIES

ANDERSON & EDNEY
Practical Animal Handling

BROWN
Aquaculture for Veterinarians: Fish Husbandry and Medicine

EMILY & PENMAN
Handbook of Small Animal Dentistry

WHITE & WILLIAMSON
The Foal

WILLS & WOLF
Handbook of Feline Medicine

Other titles of related interest

BURGER
The Waltham Book of Companion Animal Nutrition

GOLDSCHMIDT & SHOFER
Skin Tumors of the Dog and Cat

IHRKE, MASON & WHITE
Advances in Veterinary Dermatology, Volume 2

ROBINSON
Genetics for Cat Breeders, 3rd Edition
Genetics for Dog Breeders, 2nd Edition

THORNE
The Waltham Book of Dog and Cat Behaviour

WOLDEHIWET & RISTIC
Rickettsial and Chlamydial Diseases of Domestic Animals

Journal

Veterinary Dermatology
The official journal of the European Society of Veterinary Dermatology and the American College of Veterinary Dermatology

Contents

Preface

The authors' interest, knowledge and experience of veterinary practice management is the result of many years working with the veterinary profession in the United Kingdom and the United States.

John Sheridan is a veterinary surgeon who has spent many years developing and running a number of small animal veterinary practices. He is a Past President of the British Small Animal Veterinary Association, holds a Diploma in Management Studies and is an Associate of the Institute of Management Consultants. Since retiring from clinical veterinary practice in 1985 he has provided a wide range of management consultancy services for the veterinary profession and for a number of commercial organisations providing goods and services to the profession.

Owen McCafferty is a CPA who has, since 1976, devoted his entire professional efforts to the provision of tax, accounting and practice management services for the veterinary profession. In 1986 he received the Ohio Veterinary Medical Associations Meritorious Service Award and in 1988, he received the award of the American Animal Hospital Association. Owen McCafferty has written numerous tax and practice management articles and has spoken extensively within and beyond the United States. Presently he is President of the Veterinary Hospital Managers Association.

This book has been written as a contribution to the continuing development of the business of veterinary practice and to veterinary practice as a business. The authors' international views are founded in two separate professional disciplines and continental perspectives and provide a unique outlook quite different from any other veterinary practice management work yet published.

The authors have not dealt with specific countries' fiscal and statutory issues affecting veterinarians in practice. Similarities exist but the many differences could cause too much confusion. Likewise they have not dwelt on specific ethical topics which will be subject to the different requirements of a number of professional bodies nor on detailed specialty areas such as the design of veterinary practice premises and the selection and management of real estate.

Few of the ideas incorporated here are totally original and many thoughts have been inspired by clients and professional colleagues. The authors have contributed their own particular commentary on the overall theme of veterinary practice management but they wish to acknowledge with gratitude the collective contributions of a great many colleagues, writers and speakers on veterinary practice management matters. It would be quite impossible to identify specific ideas with a specific source but the authors wish to express their thanks to them all. We express our gratitude in particular to:

Susan E. Beach EA, Nick Blackwell BVSc MRCVS, John Bower BVSc MRCVS, Ian Bowley MRCVS, Peter Burgess MA VetMB MRCVS, Christine Carlson MRCVS, Thomas Catanzaro DVM MHA, Rex Chandler MA VetMB MRCVS, Ross Clark DVM, Chris Dimberline BVetMed MRCVS, Tony Cowie BVSc BSc MRCVS, Donald R. Dooley, Phil Farber DVM, John Gripper BSc MRCVS, Dixon Gunn BVMS MRCVS, Denys Harries MRCVS, William Jackson DVM MS DCVOpthal DCVSurg, Michael Kovsky DVM, Bob Levoy, Jack Marsden MICM BIM IMC, Dennis McCurnin DVM MS, Rex Nash DVM, Mark Opperman, Gordon Richards BVetMed MRCVS, James H Rosenberger DVM, Jerry Shank DVM, Gerry Snyder VMD, Geoff Startup BSc PhD DVOpthal MRCVS, John Velardo, James Wilson DVM JD, Mark Wilson BVSc MRCVS and James M Wishart MIM.

Our own practices' staffs have patiently assisted us in the composition of this work and have provided us with the available time to complete our endeavour. We thank particularly Rosemarie Guest and Simon Hughes in the UK and Mary A Light in the USA for their untiring efforts and perpetually cheerful attitude in readily accepting all the unreasonable tasks that we have asked of them.

Finally and most importantly, we dedicate this book, with thanks and love to our wives, Maureen and Colleen for their immeasurable contribution of support and encouragement.

John P. Sheridan
Owen E. McCafferty

1

A Strategy for Success

As we approached the task of writing this book, the developed world was continuing to suffer from the impact of a recession which had existed for more than two years and had a major impact on private sector manufacturing and service industries. The remaining years of the twentieth century will, in economic terms, be very different from the period of rapid growth of the 1980s. Consumers are changing. They are more cautious yet more demanding. They have more choice, and they recognize that the 1990s will be a good time to be a customer who has money to spend. For suppliers, the task will be increasingly concerned with identifying what customers seek, supplying quality goods, and developing an overriding aim of providing value for money.

Many veterinarians in practice have been facing increasing pressure on their working capital resources. Profits for many have declined and others have learned the hard way that failure to appreciate the importance of managing cashflow can be catastrophic. On the other hand very many veterinary practices continue to be extremely successful and the veterinary press throughout the world is full of reports of those practice principals who have decided 'to opt out of the recession'.

One thing seems clear: when the marketplace is allowed to function freely, consumers will be the winners in the long term. As members serving a very special caring profession we have unique ethical responsibilities to our clients and then our patients. Much of the advice and many of the services we offer, however, are not unique in the marketplace and the veterinary profession will have to concern itself increasingly with identifying and then seeking to satisfy the needs of its market, the animal-owning consumers it serves.

As we approach the final few years of the twentieth century, we are increasingly aware that the microcosm within which we live is much smaller than once we thought. The world is shrinking. Improved and faster communication, technology and information systems have brought together a wide range of business methods and disciplines for many of the professions. Professional boundaries are no longer as much of an issue as standards. Whilst the day-to-day skills and experience required for any profession are very different, the approach to managing the organisations which exist to deliver those services reveals many similarities and common objectives.

The purpose of this book is to explore and develop some of these similarities and to consider a multitude of different ideas in order to generate and retain additional profit. Within every culture, including the profession of veterinary medicine, ideas are developed through the Socratic exchange of discussion. The focus of this book is not to provide a homogeneous simplistic vision of life, but rather the means by which we can convert alternative options into opportunities for professional fulfilment, profit and success.

The Demands of Veterinary Practice

The educational demands of veterinary practice require much more than a qualification in veterinary medicine and surgery. Veterinarians, like all professionals, encompass an enormous range of knowledge. They have skills and experience in the humanities, sciences, arts, philosophy, languages, business and many other disciplines. No knowledge is useless. All the disciplines are interrelated and contribute to the rounded individuals required for success in veterinary practice. Veterinary employers should always look beyond the veterinary professional skills and qualifications of potential employees. Some time will be needed when interviewing to probe and discuss the candidates' attitudes to a number of topics,

1

be they political, philosophical, commercial or creative. At first sight, these may not be directly related to veterinary practice.

Veterinary clinicians are unique. They have a philosophy of life which is centred in a genuine concern and care for all creatures. A reverence and respect for animals is the constant thread for veterinary practitioners worldwide. It is the key motivational factor for students embarking on a career in veterinary medicine.

This innate respect for all life is popularly embodied in the existence and example of St Francis of Assisi. So intertwined is the image of St Francis in the fabric of veterinary medicine that many veterinarians all over the world adopt a sketch of the saint as a logo for their practice and as a graphic depiction of their practice mission statement. The British Veterinary Nursing Association is an example of a professional body which has incorporated the image of St Francis into its logo.

The dedication to the dignity of all creatures centred in a love for God and manifested through the example of St Francis also poses a difficult paradox for veterinarians and the clients they serve. The wish to care for the needs of animals is balanced with the requirements of a profit-motivated enterprise. Veterinarians and the staff they employ did not take a vow of poverty. The provision of quality veterinary care requires the investment of considerable resources. The St Francis ideal can be satisfied only if veterinary practice owners create and maintain profitable enterprises which satisfy the needs of owners, clients, staff and patients. They must also create a sufficient surplus to enable the practice to contribute to the welfare of animals whose owners are genuinely unable to pay for services in the private sector.

Specialisation

More and more veterinarians wish to extend their formal professional education in areas of specialist knowledge. Ophthalmology, derma-tology, orthopaedics, cardiology, general surgery, oncology, radiology and dentistry are just some examples. We are sure that a substantial demand for veterinarians with specialist clinical knowledge and

expertise will continue well into the twenty-first century. The level of income which they are able to achieve will depend on their ability to satisfy the needs of the market and of those referring veterinarians with sufficient clients who are willing and able to spend premium fees for premium advice. Increasingly, it will not just be the quality of the professional expertise which is important but the level of support services that go with it. A number of specialists have been able to establish group referral practices which can offer a range of specialist consultancy services to many first-opinion veterinary practices in the locality. We believe that the role of specialists in the private sector will continue to expand and excel when faced with competition that is steeped in bureaucratic ritual. Private specialty groups will become formidable competitors to the traditional institutional providers of specialist services.

Is the Veterinary Profession Successful?

There is an enormous body of scientific evidence which confirms the success of the veterinary profession in understanding, diagnosing and treat-ing the wide range of clinical problems which have had such a devastating impact on the economics of animal husbandry and management and the welfare of the animals involved. Many millions of animal owners have good reason to thank the veterinary profession for the unsurpassed level of professionalism, dedication and care shown by their veterinary advisers.

There is, however, plenty of evidence that all is not well in many veterinary practices. Highly qualified professional and support staff members are all too often overworked and underpaid. Too many practice principals discover that they are so 'successful' that they are overwhelmed by the volume of the tasks for which they are responsible. Could you be one of them?

Are You a Success?

- Are you in control of your practice or has it grown so fast that you are shackled by your own success?

- Is there a pile of unanswered letters, patient cards, laboratory reports and radiographs on your desk at the end of the day?
- Do you often work late to catch up with some of those outstanding tasks?
- Do you seem to have too little time to discuss cases with colleagues, attend local professional meetings or take part in continuing education programmes?
- Do you neglect your family or your hobbies?
- Do you have time to relax completely?
- Do you always seem to be short of time?
- Do you feel swamped by details?
- Do you sometimes feel stale in your professional skills?
- Are you worried by the amount of work you have to do?
- Are you bad tempered?

Perhaps you should think a bit harder and work a bit less. Spend a little of your precious time planning the way forward. If lack of time is one of your major problems, invest a little of it now to sit back, contemplate the problem, ask yourself why, and explore the opportunities for an alternative approach.

Factors for Success

What are some of the factors which separate a successful veterinary practice from the others? Is it a question of effective practice management, or the provision of the highest standards of professional service, or both? If by management we include planning strategies, setting targets, organising all the resources at our disposal and monitoring the results of our efforts, then the answer is probably 'yes, effective management does lead to success'. On the other hand there are a number of apparently well managed practices in which the principal or partners are still over-worked and under-rewarded.

The problems we have described are certainly not confined to members of the veterinary profession but are typical of the situation facing most professionals and many people in small businesses. They are hardworking and dedicated to providing a quality service for their clients, patients or customers but they sometimes fail because the management tasks overwhelm them. Standards slip. Cash becomes scarce. Physically, mentally and emotionally, they may become overloaded to the point that ill health forces closure.

We have designed this work as a practical handbook so let us try to be practical. Is it possible to identify any factors which are common to all small businesses, including the business of veterinary practice, and which predispose to failure? If we could identify some of them we would be better placed to make a start at putting things right.

What is the secret of success? What do successful business people know that the unsuccessful ones do not? The likely answer is 'plenty' but that probably has little to do with their success. Perhaps your practice reflects what you are. If you are sloppy your practice will be sloppy; if you are innovative so will be your practice; if you are positive and confident your practice will similarly be perceived as positive.

Your practice is a professional enterprise which must function profitably in a business environment. Effective business activity and the pursuit of professional standards are not mutually exclusive but rather inclusive. Veterinary practices cannot survive in the 1990s and beyond without equitable attention being devoted to the skill, ethics and the business of medicine and surgery. Good medicine is good for business. In turn financial success generates the resources necessary to purchase the medical and surgical equipment and up-to-date veterinary facilities which are necessary to offer quality professional services and veterinary medicine.

Most veterinary practice owners are dedicated, knowledgeable and enthusiastic clinicians but many are reluctant practice managers. Perhaps the mistake we make is in assuming that an understanding of the technical aspects of the business of veterinary medicine is an adequate qualification for understanding the nature of a business that provides veterinary services. Increasingly we are sure that **this is simply not true.**

The Professional in Business

The professional services provided by a veterinary practice require a wide range of professional skills, experience and expertise. The business of delivering veterinary skills and services in the marketplace demands quite a different set of attributes. For many, perhaps the majority of practising veterinarians, the practice is not a business but a place where they can practice their profession.

Why then do veterinarians become practice owners or partners in a veterinary practice? Because they don't want to work for other people any longer? Because they will be better off financially? Or maybe because they can practice their profession in premises and in a style which suits them. Their profession is their vocation; they become absorbed with furthering their understanding and education in a specific area of interest; they like buying veterinary gadgets and in developing new diagnostic or surgical techniques. Veterinarians are great enthusiasts for their profession.

Most small businesses are established by skilled artisans, technicians or professionals; hairdressers, house decorators, dressmakers, accountants, physicians, architects, builders, dentists, mechanics and veterinarians. All are human beings who go into business on their own account. They are a mixture of three people: the visionary entrepreneur, the organising manager and the skilled expert. Each separate personality wants to take the lead. When there is a conflict between them, the professional expert will nearly always win simply because the proprietor is usually a trained professional. This may be very good for the professional but is probably very bad for the business. The three skills are like the legs of a tripod. If they were well balanced the business would have an inherent strength to cope with the financial, social and other pressures which face any small business. Unfortunately the skills are not evenly balanced in any one individual and in veterinary practice a typical breakdown might be: professional 70%, entrepreneur 20%, manager 10%.

Professional, Entrepreneur or Manager?

Who are these three personalities in the world of veterinary practice? The entrepreneur is the visionary, the dreamer who is always living for the future but for whom the dull routine of actually running the practice is frankly irksome. As long as the dream is attainable, the visionary will function in the present but covet the future.

The manager is the pragmatist. If there were no manager there would be no planning, no order and no predictability. The manager is the organiser; he or she sees the problem, identifies what has happened in the past and attempts to create order out of chaos. The manager's nature is to pursue predictability through systems of control.

The veterinarian is the professional: the professional is the doer. If a technical job needs to be done, the professional will get on and do it. The doer enjoys his or her profession; veterinary practice is his or her hobby. He or she is an individualist and is determined not to be part of a disciplined system. He or she treasures the elegance of the art of practice.

To the manager in veterinary practice, the veterinarian becomes a problem to be controlled. To the veterinarian, the manager becomes a bureaucratic meddler to be avoided and to the entrepreneur, the manager and the veterinarian are precious resources who are recruited to deal with the chore of working for today to accommodate tomorrow.

Leadership and Management

We need to distinguish between that which could be and that which is. Management by its very definition is concerned with quantifying, moulding and monitoring resources which already exist. Leadership on the other hand requires a vision. It is the basis upon which an organisation meets the challenges of the day and those of the future.

Balance must be accommodated. The issue is one of potential versus actual. Visionaries contemplate the potential; management limits the actual. Leaders actuate the potential. Ongoing success depends crucially on a generous measure of each. Leaders in the business of veterinary practice keep an eye on the present whilst seeking a vision of the future. The interplay between good management and astute vision is a balance of both these objectives through effective, dynamic leadership.

Proper leadership demands a body of knowledge, a set of standards, and a commitment to a vision. In veterinary practice, the body of knowledge must be founded on a strong base of professional and clinical understanding and expertise, on sound financial practices, on a sensitive understanding of the needs of those who work in the practice and on an awareness of the dynamics of the marketplace and the patients served.

Within many practice environments, leadership and management have been confused. Two distinct issues must be followed: Camelot and Constantinople. Camelot, the kingdom that might have been, and Constantinople, the old world symbol of pragmatic trade, must be merged like the ideal and the reality. If there is a single need that outweighs all others, it is the need for vision counterbalanced by the discipline for sticking to the rules. This balance must be addressed realistically and consistently to satisfy the demands of a vibrant, progressive, innovative, profitable and growing practice.

The leader has a responsibility to ensure that the organisation is managed methodically and consistently. The visionary may not be an appropriate manager. Vision without management is not leadership. Management without vision results in mindless compliance. Leadership balances these two extremes.

What is Their Secret?

The principals of successful practices seem to have a high profile. Successful principals do their homework; they formulate a plan, formally or informally. They feel very strongly about the philosophy of the practice. They lead by example and ensure that every single member of the practice is aware of that philosophy and feels part of it. Very often successful practices appear to be led by a principal or partners who work fewer hours and yet achieve a significantly higher level of income.

There is nothing new about 'practice management' but perhaps the level of management expertise which resulted in success in the past is no longer sufficient. The world in which we practice is changing. Donald Dooley, a successful management consultant to veterinary practice in the United States has said that 'there are three types of veterinarians — those who make things happen, those who watch things happen and those who wonder "What the hell happened!"'

Pearls of Wisdom

On the assumption that you are a veterinary surgeon or practice manager who is intent on making things happen, are there any pearls of wisdom worth bearing in mind? Most management consultants believe you should:

- Take advice judiciously. Trust yet verify.
- Stick to what you know and know what you are sticking to.
- Plan with flexibility. Understand the dynamic continuum of practice management.
- Delegate — don't be indispensable.
- Introduce information systems and follow through diligent monitoring.
- Never underestimate the importance of service. Satisfied clients validate practice worth.
- Don't take out too much too soon. Conserve capital.
- Communicate with your partners, your staff and your clients.
- Don't forget your family.
- Manage your cashflow and profitability.
- Manage your time and encourage your associates to follow your lead.
- Lead by example, not dictum.
- Set clear objectives.
- Enjoy it while it lasts; savour the moment.
- Make service your obsession.
- Have a business plan. Update and revise it regularly. Use it.

Good Ethics are Good for Business

A profession by its very nature demands a code of ethics and a body of knowledge. For members of the veterinary profession, both are demanding and comprehensive. The formal written code is usually prepared and modified by the appropriate professional body as necessary and as circumstances change. The Guide to Professional Conduct published by the Royal College of

Veterinary Surgeons in the United Kingdom, for example, includes the following note: 'Some people would say that ethical guidance and rulings as to professional conduct are set out solely for the purpose of controlling the non conformists to be found in any profession. But this is rather a negative view to take. In every civilized society people have to put their heads together to prepare a code of law or to record recognised customs which they are prepared to follow in order to ensure the stability of the state and thus ensure their own freedom to go about their business without always having to look over their shoulders to see what their neighbours are up to. In agreeing to this, men, of course, surrender a measure of their individual liberty in return for the assurance that it will no longer be open to those neighbours to do entirely as they please regardless of the effect of such conduct upon others. Experience has shown that in societies where no rules are laid down or observed and the popular sentiment has been that the devil may take the hindmost, the devil hasn't stopped at the hindmost. He has devoured them all.'

In addition to the written formal code most individual professionals superimpose their own personal ethical standards over and above those required by their profession. The formal code of conduct then becomes regarded as a baseline standard of professional behaviour.

Some believe that the only way to satisfy the profession's code of ethics is to wait for clients to contact the practice and to deal with specific problems as and when requested. Professional responsibilities for the interests of patients can only be adequately discharged by policies designed to seek out undiagnosed and untreated departures from health and to offer vigorous and positive advice about the preventive, diagnostic, medical, surgical or other measures necessary to deal with them. If, for example, professional clinical judgement determines a specific course of action for a particular case, a failure positively to recommend such action may be considered as a breach of veterinary ethical requirements.

Ethics become a critical issue when the morality of practice is discussed. At practice level, one of the most important leadership roles may be to monitor employee practitioners to ensure that professional quality and ethical standards are being maintained. The public, as consumers of veterinary services, assume a certain code of conduct and expect a level of fair dealing with the veterinary profession.

Sadly, within any profession ethical standards are sometimes breached. The veterinary profession is no exception. Veterinarians have been known to charge for procedures that have not been performed or to perform those procedures on patients which are already dead. Harsh handling of patients, and insensitive or inadequate communication with clients are perhaps more common sins. Clients expect and demand the highest level of empathy by the veterinarian towards the patient and generally the veterinary profession has a reputation for conducting itself at a standard which is unparalleled by any other animal health care provider.

Continuing Professional Development

A commitment to being the best demands the greatest effort. Dedication to continuing education (continuing professional development) is a minimum requirement for those clinicians who are committed to providing a quality level of service. Thoughtful reading becomes an essential element of the practice of veterinary medicine. Professional journals, text books, video tapes, audio tapes, continuing professional education courses and Socratic professional exchanges with colleagues are some of the methods that help to sharpen the clinician's knowledge base.

Experience is a wonderful teacher but experience alone is not enough. Experience gained does not always reflect lessons learned. Formalised education in the form of short courses, university or commercially sponsored seminars, in-practice staff training sessions, articles written either for the general public or for colleagues' professional publications, and papers delivered to client groups and to practice or professional colleagues all help veterinarians to establish a standard of personal excellence.

Consider planning your own personal syllabus for continuing professional development. Commit yourself to establishing and building upon a personal level of expertise in a particular area of practice which you find particularly challenging. You should plan to devote at least one hour a day to your chosen special interest and you will be amazed at how much it will help you to enjoy every aspect of the day-to-day routine of clinical practice. There will be a cost in time and resources and we recommend that you allocate a specific and adequate part of your budget as a percentage of practice revenue to finance the books, the subscriptions, the courses, travel, meals and subsistence which will be needed if you and your staff are to make the best of the continuing education possibilities which exist. Keep a chronicle of your study and a commentary of your observations by maintaining a diary. Writing forces reflection. Your own endeavours in professional development are documented and customised to your own needs and capabilities. Use study as a tool to generate profit. The knowledge you gain may be converted into new or improved professional services. You may keep a second journal for practice management issues. Encourage associates to follow your lead. Swap journals and seek exchange learning with professional colleagues inside and outside the practice. A fresh viewpoint of a revolutionary idea may be the needed perspective to convert the theory into profitable practice.

At a minimum, we believe that 0.75% to 1.5% of gross income should be devoted to a practice's continuing education budget. Your clients should be aware of your practice's commitment to obtaining the latest technical and professional information. You need to satisfy their demands for professional excellence.

Every single member of your staff should be exposed to and have an opportunity of participating in continuing professional development. If you have selected them wisely, your professional and support staff will also commit themselves to provide the quality level of service that you demand. Their base of knowledge must also be expanded and nurtured through professional development.

Your staff have been attracted to veterinary medicine for many reasons other than monetary gain. If you doubt that, have another look at their pay cheques. They are dedicated people who invest a great deal of their lives to the interests of veterinary medicine and animal welfare. The best will be attracted to those practices committed to providing regular continuing education for their employees. At all levels, continuing education generates employees' interests in their positions. The benefits will accrue for you, your clients and your patients.

Management Education

Practice management issues also require a basis of knowledge which needs to be reinforced and maintained by a comprehensive programme of continuing education. An image for quality in the delivery of medical and surgical veterinary services must be matched by a similar level of competence, efficiency and quality in the ways in which the practice conducts its business. Everybody involved in running a veterinary practice is involved in managing something or someone. Those skills must constantly be exercised and honed to be effective. Whenever possible, encourage your practice manager or other management staff to belong to any appropriate professional associations which may exist, such as the Veterinary Hospital Managers Association in Canada and the United States. In North America, the American Animal Hospital Association and the Veterinary Hospital Managers Association are developing certification programmes for practice managers. In the United Kingdom, a number of commercial and professional organisations provide a range of seminars and other training programs for reception, bookkeeping, communication and other management skills.

In our experience, veterinary practice support staff members are generally willing, able and enthusiastic to be very much more actively involved in the management of the practice resources to achieve the success that they, and you, seek. The role of practice manager has evolved into a profession with a distinct body of knowledge and code of ethics. Accordingly, the practice manager's professional knowledge must also be renewed and updated through continuing education and by developing associations with colleagues facing similar professional challenges at home and overseas.

Summary

A strategy for successful veterinary practice in the 1990s and early in the new century should include:

- An obsession with the provision of quality professional services and a commitment to the highest ethical standards.
- A thirst for leadership and a determination to ensure that every member of the practice is involved in managing practice resources effectively and efficiently.
- A long-term investment in continuing professional development in all the clinical and non-clinical skills which your practice will need if it is to achieve the objectives you seek.

2

Management in a Veterinary Setting

Large multi-partner veterinary practices or groups involving a number of partners and employing veterinarians, veterinary nurses, technicians and trainees and reception, clerical and other support staff are still very small enterprises by comparison with the generally accepted definition of small businesses. Whether practices are run by sole proprietors, partnerships or as legal corporate entities, the practice owners are intimately involved in determining practice policies and in implementing the measures designed to achieve them. Practice principals find it difficult to separate practice objectives from personal and professional dreams and ambitions.

Successful practices are run by happy staff. Whole books have been written to identify the source of staff happiness. Most would agree that the attributes which contribute to a measure of personnel happiness would include at least some of the following:

- Peace of mind implying freedom from fear, guilt and anger.
- Good health and the energy to enjoy an active life.
- Good personal relationships with others.
- Freedom from financial worries.
- Feelings of personal fulfilment.
- Worthy and achievable goals and objectives and a sense of being in charge of one's own life.

Successful practices enable practice directors to achieve at least some of those attributes. Veterinary practice principals will increasingly recognise the importance of keeping abreast of practice management developments, in addition to their investment in technical and professional expertise and innovation.

The management methods you used last year may have produced a satisfactory level of return. The same may not be true today. These techniques will become increasingly inadequate. Next year and the year after they may become positively antiquated. Consumers are changing. They are better informed, more demanding, more selective, increasingly concerned with quality and value for money and have a greater choice.

The Management Role

The management role is a very wide one but in essence it encompasses:

- Planning — the setting of objectives.
- Organising — acquiring and managing the resources required to achieve those objectives. These will include staff, premises, equipment, stock and finance.
- Control — the establishment of monitoring procedures designed to ensure that policies are being implemented and that targets are being achieved.

Every member of the practice team is concerned with management. The reception staff manage the computer terminal, the record cards, the day books and appointment arrangements. Clinical and nursing staff must manage the in-patient facilities, the drugs and dressings, the surgical instruments and equipment and the patients. The practice manager, the office manager, the head nurse or the secretary may be responsible for managing all personnel matters, and the practice owner, principal or partners are ultimately responsible for the management of all the practice assets to ensure that they are used effectively, efficiently and economically to achieve the practice objectives.

The overall practice managerial role includes responsibility for strategic planning. Ultimately, the owners of the practice must determine practice objectives and develop a range of clinical, marketing, personnel and financial policies which are designed to achieve them. One vision must link all these disciplines.

A further important management role is to implement the wide range of administrative tasks designed to ensure that the practice runs as planned and that its policies are implemented. This will require the establishment of a system for recording and collecting the information needed for well informed decision making, in a meaningful format, as and when it is required.

A growing number of veterinary practices employ practice managers. In the United States, the Veterinary Hospital Managers Association was established to promote the importance of management skills in veterinary practice and to look after the interests of its members. The job description of the individuals involved varies widely and can extend from a senior support staff member, whose responsibilities have been extended to include a number of administrative tasks, to individuals with personnel, management or accountancy training who are responsible to the principals for the efficient conduct of every aspect of practice activity.

Who are the Managers?

Veterinarians

Semi- or complete retirement from clinical practice is achieved by some practice owners who accept an alternative job function within the practice. The most cost-effective role for any experienced clinician is as a veterinarian rather than as a manager. Accepting a full-time management position in veterinary medicine is not the best use of the skill and the knowledge of an experienced veterinarian but it may be seen as a way in which a particular individual might retain an important advisory role in the practice without the burden of nights and weekends on duty as a clinician. Younger colleagues might regard such a role for a senior partner as being the worst of all worlds. They will not appreciate a manager whom they perceive as seeking to restrict their freedom to implement the innovative and fundamental policy measures they believe necessary. At the same time, the senior adviser is not generating

the level of practice income which was possible before his or her 'retirement'.

Veterinary practice management may be a viable alternative for veterinarians who no longer wish to practice their profession as clinicians. They must appreciate, however, that the level of remuneration they might expect will probably be significantly lower than that they would achieve as practising veterinarians. There are however, some examples of veterinarians who have taken on a full-time role to manage a number of separate practices on behalf of their owners. In such cases it may be that their knowledge, skills and expertise could result in the design and implementation of new business systems which might generate enhanced levels of profit and thus justify a salary level comparable with that achieved by the owners.

The most important function in a veterinary practice is the practice of veterinary medicine. Management is a critical additional role but it is a separate and a supportive one. We believe that for practices of any size, individuals with sufficient background knowledge of veterinary practice and the skills required to carry out practice management tasks can be recruited at a far lower cost than that of an experienced veterinarian. If a clinical veterinarian is competent and capable of practicing veterinary medicine, their most cost-effective use is by practicing their profession. The veterinarian could and most certainly should still exhibit the necessary leadership as practice principal, but does not have to devote his or her full time and effort to a management position.

The management function is to carry out the policies of the practice owners using the available resources in the most effective manner to achieve the objectives specified. Depending on the precise specification of the job and the individual's level of experience, a veterinary manager will probably need far less supervision than, for example, a new veterinary graduate.

Support Staff

Veterinary nurses, technicians and other support staff can no longer be regarded simplistically as individuals with a particular clinical skill or expertise whose contribution to overall practice activity is limited to that expertise. Many of them are keen to look beyond their own present level of knowledge and are enthusiastic to expand their involvement and to take a positive and active role in helping to manage the enterprise in which they work. Wise employers will further encourage that interest by investing time and money in them and assist these associate managers to hone their skills in the interests of a long-term, mutually beneficial relationship.

A wide variety of part- and full-time continuing education courses and seminars are available for reception, clerical, bookkeeping and administrative staff. If individual needs are carefully matched with the course material available, the individuals will be provided with a firm basis in understanding the business of veterinary medicine and expanding the scope of their knowledge and their level of remuneration.

This base of knowledge is not only good for the staff member but also for the practice. One of the most important leadership roles is to spot those promising individuals with a flare for excellence and offer them career opportunities beyond the scope of their present level of service.

Managers may be described as caretakers of a well organised garden. Their function is to maintain, prune, and nurture whilst accepting that, frequently, influences beyond their control may have a critical part to play in their efforts to succeed. A good veterinary practice manager understands the analogy. We live in a hapless environment where chance can become a good friend or a continual adversary. Change, by its very nature, demands a creative positive response. Those involved in determining the direction of the practice determine the course but leave the day-to-day control of the rudder to the practice manager.

Personnel management is only one of the skills required. Handling people effectively demands the sensitivity of a poet yet the firmness of a loving parent. A good custodial practice manager must accept the responsibility for unpleasant as well as joyous tasks. Hard work, understanding, patience, and resolution of purpose are hallmarks of a good custodial manager in a veterinary practice.

Practice managers have existed informally in practices over the last 25 to 30 years. Much confusion still exists about terminology but, gradually, the lines of delineation are becoming more clearly defined in terms of leadership versus custodianship.

The role of practice managers in veterinary medicine is evolving. Since the inception of the Veterinary Hospital Managers Association in 1981, the veterinary profession in North America has seen a dramatic increase in the demand for professional hospital managers. A greater awareness and deserved respect is now afforded to individuals who enter the profession of veterinary practice management. The VHMA has developed an examination programme to demonstrate a comprehensive body of knowledge and adhere to a standardised code of ethics.

The VHMA has included members from countries outside the United States and Canada and for the last 11 years has been actively involved in formulating the concept of worldwide practice management. The American Animal Hospital Association has also been hard at work over the last 5 years in shaping and moulding the job description and areas of responsibility for management staff in veterinary practice. Although these two North American organisations have been in the vanguard of organised practice management, many other associations and publications worldwide, have also espoused an expansive role for practice managers.

Varying skill levels are required for the range of management tasks within veterinary practice. Not only is the level of remuneration an issue, but degrees of authority, direction and competence will need to be determined. Prior experience and perceived levels of knowledge and responsibility by other members of staff can become important in determining job titles, areas of responsibility and pay. Matching work with worth is not easy. A natural human tendency exists to offer a title and level of remuneration which exceeds that which the level of competence demands. Negotiation of such issues becomes crucial in managing the development of administrative personnel who seek to extend their careers into veterinary office or practice management.

The following titles and job descriptions are

becoming readily accepted in practice in the United States and Canada and are offered as a pattern for the profession elsewhere.

The Office Manager

Office managers may be regarded as the first level of veterinary practice management. Their role is to help implement and coordinate the administrative directions determined by the practice owner or hospital director. Leadership by the practice principal or hospital director becomes the basis upon which the office manager responds. The position of office manager is generally the first step on the ladder which leads to the post of veterinary hospital administrator.

The office manager will be responsible for the effective implementation of routine office tasks. The office manager originally may have been a receptionist, nurse, technician or clerical staff member who was responsible for making appointments, paying accounts, posting receipts and payments, banking, interviewing personnel, ordering drugs and other stock and preparing pay-rolls. Sometimes the office manager's role evolves from tasks initially carried out by bookkeepers who become skilled in veterinary terminology and promoted to positions of trust and responsibility. In some instances, administrative assistants or secretaries have earned the position of office manager, whilst in other practices the role of administrative assistant, who may be a personal assistant to the practice principal or hospital administrator, may be senior to the office manager.

Successful office managers can thus evolve from a variety of disciplines and the skills required are primarily administrative and organisational in nature. They require a clear understanding of the philosophy as well as of the practical routine inherent in a veterinary practice.

The office manager's skills demand a level of knowledge which includes not only business management but also a firm grasp of psychology and a level of competence and confidence in man management. In employment issues, for example, the office manager may be the individual who has the skill, experience, and common sense necessary to deal with the tricky personnel problems which arise in all organisations from time to time. It is

clear that the personnel role, encompassing as it does recruitment, retention and training issues, will be of increasing importance.

It may be the office manager who will be responsible for such matters as coordinating the ordering of drugs and professional supplies, summarising receipts and payments or working with the practice's accountant or management consultant to complete the books and records or to prepare management accounting and other data. Depending on the size of the enterprise, the office manager may or may not personally prepare the figures but will certainly be responsible for coordinating and collating the various specific tasks involved. Managers will be responsible for understanding the need for data generated by manual and computerised systems and the discipline required to retrieve and utilise it productively.

The Practice Manager

The second skill level seen in practice is that of practice manager. Generally the practice manager's responsibilities are greater than that of an office manager and may include the overall coordination of financial activities, preparation of budgets, maintaining personnel records, and evaluating all the practice employees including veterinarians, technicians, nurses, clerical and other support staff.

The practice manager's role may also include planning, coordinating and recommending policies as well as strategic issues for debate and consideration by the equity owners of the practice. The principal or partners will make the broad policy decisions and have the ultimate veto power over every segment of practice activity but the practice manager, who will normally be responsible to the hospital director or to the principal, will have more authority than the office manager over the day-to-day operation of the practice and will be responsible for dismissing as well as hiring support staff.

As practice managers evolve their responsibility they may help to resolve disputes over salaries and performance-related pay policies for professional and all staff members. Practice managers will need to be skilled and sensitive communicators and will ensure that all practice personnel are provided with the information they need to carry out their responsibilities.

The role of practice manager may not be an easy one and much will depend on the perception of the role by the practice principal. Not infrequently equity owners, for example, may undermine the authority of practice managers by over-riding specific decisions that they would wish to make. Very often the owner of a veterinary practice, whilst wishing to maintain the ultimate decision-making authority, will employ a practice manager to deal with the day-to-day managerial responsibilities in the practice. Many principals are realistic enough to recognise that they are best employed as clinicians and cannot possibly oversee every administrative function but are not prepared to let go of the reigns of management completely. The role of practice manager may be regarded as a transitional step between that of office manager and hospital administrator.

The Practice or Hospital Administrator

The final tier of practice management is that of practice or hospital administrator, a role carried out by an individual who has complete authority over the day-to-day operation of the practice. The hospital director, the partners or principal, the equity holders in the practice, do not abdicate responsibility but merely allocate and authorise that responsibility.

The veterinary administrator's function is similar to that of a chief executive officer of a large corporation. The hospital administrator has the skill level to coordinate all practice activities.

Hospital administrators are most commonly found in the very largest of veterinary hospital practices. They are highly qualified and accomplished individuals who know the business of veterinary practice intimately, are widely experienced and have gained the admiration and trust of the principals who employ them. Their competence, their knowledge and their ethical standards are of the highest level and their basis of remuneration must reflect the responsibility which they bear.

The obvious limitation for the hospital admini-

strator is the willingness of the owner to relinquish the degree of authority needed to enable the administrator to function effectively. Professional hospital administration is successful only if it is allowed to be.

The practice owners, as clinicians, are clearly responsible for all the clinical standards and issues. The hospital administrator is responsible for every other aspect of practice activity and is perceived by the clients as the ultimate organiser, planner and authority figure in the practice for such matters. For all routine non-clinical purposes, the owners of the practice become employees, abdicating their day-to-day managerial responsibilities in exchange for higher incomes, fewer headaches and an enhanced quality of life.

The transition towards this abdication of authority is a substantial stumbling block for most veterinarians. The last vestige of authoritarianism in the world seems to be in ownership of a small business. Abdicating ownership rights of authority to a better qualified third party becomes a quantum leap that many practice owners simply cannot accept. Great lip service is paid to the desire to 'let go' but in reality, very few practice owners have the wisdom, confidence or capability of not interfering.

Some owners evolve a recognition that the demands of management are beyond their experience, skills or wishes. As hospitals grow in size and stature some veterinarian hospital directors may choose to give up clinical responsibilities to meet the challenge of a full-time managerial and administrative role. More commonly, the overworked principal recognises that his greatest value is in the consulting room or operating theatre.

To date, very few veterinary hospital administrators have been appointed. It might be argued that an unwillingness by owners to accept the need to hand over the degree of responsibility and authority required by a practice administrator has positively diminished the opportunity for administrators to excel. For the business of veterinary practice to rise to the level of service and profitability which is possible, trust must be exhibited in the manager by the equity owner(s).

The practice or hospital administrator will need

a clear brief to understand the constraints within which to operate. The non-veterinary manager must be positively involved in determining the overall practice mission, setting specific objectives and in establishing the control measures which will be necessary. The level of continuity needed to affect a change by a hospital administrator and the degree of administrative sophistication which is possible, are perhaps the biggest advantages of engaging a hospital administrator. The director's vision may not be that of the administrator. The director's vision can be turned into reality by the manager.

The knowledge required to be an effective practice or hospital administrator extends far beyond the disciplines of veterinary medicine and surgery. Obtaining a veterinary degree does not automatically qualify a person as hospital administrator — far from it. Indeed, we have suggested that a knowledge of the technical aspects of the business of veterinary medicine is most certainly not an adequate qualification for understanding the nature of a business that provides veterinary services. Effective veterinary practice administration is not degree-oriented but rather education-oriented.

Experienced practice managers, office managers, veterinary nurses, technicians, veterinarians or individuals recruited from outside the world of veterinary medicine can all gravitate eventually towards the knowledge base demanded of a hospital administrator. The skills required encompass a thorough understanding of a wide range of management skills including strategic planning, marketing, personnel management and financial matters. Further skills include a recognition of the commitment required to identify and provide a range of quality services sought by clients at a market price. These skills must be nurtured, developed and earned. The most important function of the hospital director, practice principal or equity owner will be to identify, recruit, recognise and retain individuals who demonstrate the potential for developing these skills.

Most veterinarians now recognise that the further they are separated from individual fee calculations, the better off they will be. Now is the time to persuade practice principals that their prime and most productive role is to concentrate on their clinical skills, determine the strategy, lead by example, have the vision, establish the standards and appoint the best office manager, practice manager or hospital administrator that they can find.

3

Planning for Success

Management is concerned with the crucial need to plan, to determine specific objectives, to organise the resources required, and to establish a monitoring system to ensure that practice policies are being implemented.

Let us look a little more closely at the first of these items — the business plan. The veterinary businesses which grow and prosper in the coming years will be those in which the practice owners have spent some of their precious time developing an intelligent, written business plan. Busy practice principals tend to defer consideration of the important, but perhaps less urgent, management issues because of the pressures of the day. The daily demands of clients about the urgent needs of their animals consume most of their time.

At 7.30am on a busy Monday, planning may not seem as urgent as the long list of demanding clients and patients which must be seen before lunch. Planning may not be so urgent but it is most certainly just as important. It doesn't matter too much whether you start to plan now or tomorrow or next week. The problem is that if you leave it until next week you may never get started at all. Planning takes time. Even with a plan you won't get it right all the time. You can be sure however, that practices which plan the way ahead get it mostly right most of the time.

Success for any veterinary practice in this rapidly changing world will depend as always on professional ability, communication skills, hard work, tenacity, enthusiasm, flexibility, imagination, determination to succeed and leadership. To these we must now add the ability and the will to plan. It has been said that 'failing to plan' positively implies 'planning to fail'.

Planning in Practice

Consider the following questions:

WHY? — Why should you prepare a plan for your practice?

Peter Drucker, management guru and author, confirms that time is a professional's scarcest resource. Effective practice principals and managers know where their time goes. They set priorities and stay with them. Focusing on those activities which bring results, veterinarians concentrate on their strengths to achieve their objectives. An ounce of implementation is worth a ton of philosophy. Implementation requires a plan.

WHEN? — When do you need to prepare a plan?

When you set up or purchase a practice, when you take on a partner or purchase a partnership, when you perceive a need for a change of direction or emphasis and as part of an ongoing review as the practice develops and when you want to borrow money, you must plan.

The planning process is as important for the solo veterinarian setting up, purchasing or continuing to run an established practice as it is for the principal(s) of a large multi-person, multi-premises organisation. No one is immune from the need.

Remember too that effective planning is not a process of merely rolling forward last year's accounts and adding 'a bit for inflation'. It is a question of taking a long hard look at the things you want to do over the next three to five years and setting out the steps you will need to take and the resources you will require to do them.

WHO? — Who will be interested in the plan?

Partners and potential partners as the investors in the enterprise; those who manage and run the practice — your staff and those who lend money to the practice (bank managers, finance companies, insurance companies and other sources of capital) will all be interested. Lenders of significant capital sums will certainly want to know:

- How much you want to borrow?

- What you want it for?
- When and how you plan to repay the principal.
- What security you can offer.

They will want to be satisfied that you can repay both the principal and interest and they will want to see that you could survive a set-back in plans.

You and your fellow investors will also want to know the answers to those questions. Identify where you are now, where you want to go, how you propose to get there and be sure that the whole enterprise is worthwhile. In short, a comprehensive business plan will enable you to test the potential financial viability of the practice.

WHAT? — What will the plan comprise?

Most definitions of management include setting objectives, identifying and organising the resources required, and establishing control measures to monitor performance.

Your business plan therefore should attempt to answer the following questions:

- Can you express your practice philosophy (mission statement) and the broad practice strategy verbally and in writing?
- Is there a common understanding amongst the partners about shared personal and practice values?
- Are those values understood and appreciated by your staff and your clients?
- Is your spouse in accord with your strategy?
- What is the nature of the practice now?
- Can you identify what the practice is doing right and what it could be doing much better, its strengths and weaknesses?
- What trends have you observed during the last couple of years?
- What is happening in the world beyond the immediate practice locality?
- What changes are occurring in your catchment area and what influence could they have on your practice?
- What problems, opportunities and challenges are you facing now or expect to face shortly?
- What personal and practice objectives do you want to set for the next two years?

- What resources will you need and what will you have to do to achieve them and how will you know when you have done so?

Later sections of this book will deal in much greater detail with financial, marketing and personnel planning but for now let us begin to prepare a skeleton planning document which we can flesh out later.

The Strategic Plan

The successful conduct of a veterinary practice demands vision, leadership skills and a clear definition of the practice's mission statement. A practice is the embodiment of the dreams and aspirations of the owner veterinarian. The practice image, its perception in the eyes of professional colleagues, the staff, the clients and others in the locality is determined by the individual character and values of the owner. As the practice evolves, many other individuals become involved. Procedures and systems change and original staff members are inevitably replaced by new faces. Slowly but surely, the original practice image may fade. Unless determined steps are taken by the owner(s) to redefine and reaffirm the practice philosophy and the values by which it operates, there is a danger of decline and decay. The practice must be steered positively along a planned course of development by a leader with the necessary vision for the future.

On a sheet of paper try to define the nature of your practice as it is now. Identify in writing the services it offers, the premises it occupies and the personnel it employs. What is special, what is unique about your practice?

Why should any animal owner in the vicinity seek advice from your practice rather than from your competitors? Do you know for sure that the image of you, your staff and your practice in the area is the image you would wish to have? Now note down those key features of your existing clients and patients and the problems which they present which you can and do satisfy. What about those needs which you cannot or choose not to satisfy?

Talk the statement over with your colleagues and your staff. What's changing whether you like it or not? What would you like to change and what opportunities exist to help you make those changes?

The Mission

Use those preliminary notes to prepare a statement — a strategic mission statement — which will identify your practice as you wish it to be in two years time. A mission statement is simply a clear and concise statement incorporating that vision and the means by which it will be achieved. The vision is the ideal. Short- or medium-term objectives are determined on the basis of what can realistically be achieved in that timeframe. Fulfilling those objectives will bring the practice closer to the ideal. The ideal may never be achieved but the vision it encompasses must be stated and restated. Given time and consistency, the mission statement will be reflected in the practice image. Management's role is to ensure that the perceived image is close to the owner's ideal. A tendency exists for the mission statement to be a wordy expression of everything a practitioner thinks should be said rather than the heartfelt expression of where the practice is going. The mission statement is more than simply a target. It must include an identification of the market to be served, the services to be offered, the resources which will be required and the characteristics which will make the business unique.

The following is a simple example:

"The mission of the Achill Island Animal Hospital is to provide a comprehensive range of first opinion preventive, diagnostic, medical and surgical veterinary services for the owners of domestic pet animals in a geographical area within a ten mile radius of the hospital. The market segment we serve will comprise all those owners who demand and are prepared to pay for a high-quality, caring and compassionate service. The income generated ensures a healthy level of investment in premises, equipment and training for every member of staff. The professional and support staff are paid significantly more than the average in the locality but their level of dedication and commitment to quality is also high. We endeavour to meet the professional and service needs of our clients and their animals promptly and, wherever possible, to exceed their expectations. Our overriding philosophy is to offer a unique, quality, caring, professional service at fee levels which are perceived as 'costly but excellent value for money".

That statement embodies a whole series of budgetary requirements. The practice will not undercut but will charge fee levels designed to ensure that practice employees and owners receive just compensation for their level of professionalism. The statement implies an on-going level of investment in the best equipment, the most complete drug inventory, and the most meticulous attention to the maintenance and operation of practice services. No effort will be spared in order to accomplish the mission. The mission statement specifically refers to the needs of the client as well as their pets. The practice is consumer rather than service oriented. The mission demands that the practice will only employ dedicated, hard-working, enthusiastic, highly motivated and highly paid staff. The mission statement identifies a companion animal practice and it is clear that the owner(s) have made a conscious deliberate decision to exclude large animal or equine patients. It recognises that no practice can please all the people all the time and the owner has decided to concentrate the best possible level of service to a specific market segment.

The statement can be a lengthy, multi-claused declaration or a series of short sentences. It must be known, understood and accepted by every single member of the practice and it must be truthful, accurate and realistic.

The idea of a mission statement has probably been overused by a plethora of practice management consultants. Effectively used, the mission statement becomes the primary tool for direction in the practice. The exercise requires input from all key personnel. The final determination of practice direction resides with the practice leadership, that is the equity owner with the greatest risk, but considered input by personnel in all departments is crucial. The owner will come to recognise that in the best planned and managed practices, personnel come and go but the leadership remains.

The more specific you can be, the more likely

you are to achieve your objectives. The statement will need to be fairly detailed and should include:

- The precise nature of the services you offer.
- Special features which make your practice unique.
- Who are your clients and where do they come from?
- Identify your patients by species and by the clinical problems they represent?
- What are your specific objectives relating to service development, employees, growth, turnover, profits and case volume?
- The premises and facilities you will need to provide those services.
- What staff numbers and skills you will require.

Once you have written the first draft statement, fix an opportunity to discuss it again with your colleagues and prepare a revised and refined version.

In a well planned and well managed practice, the mission statement and the financial reality will coincide. A high-quality practice with a low fee structure will eventually not be commercially viable. A practice with a blended balance between objectives and resources will rarely result in that malady which affects many veterinary practice owners and which is commonly referred to as 'burnout'. The message for practice principals, partners, owners and directors who no longer find veterinary practice challenging and fun, is to take time out to rethink their professional values and aspirations, prepare a mission statement and turn it into reality by preparing and implementing a practice plan.

Finally, the mission statement must be utilised. It must be referred to frequently. It must be posted in a prominent position for everyone to see. It must be reexamined and updated when necessary and formal steps for review involving all the members of staff should be undertaken on a regular basis, at least annually, to ensure that the promise embodied in the mission statement is being delivered.

Defining, agreeing and refining the mission statement is only the beginning. The owners,

the veterinarians, the technicians, the nursing, reception and clerical staff — everybody associated with the practice — must shoulder some degree of responsibility to ensure that the promise of its lofty ideals is delivered.

The Financial Plan

The next stage is to prepare a financial statement which identifies the current financial position, summarises financial performance over the previous three years, and identifies the practice financial strengths and weaknesses. Consider your broad approach to your financial plan. Make some value judgements about some or all of the following parameters (they are discussed in greater detail in Chapter 7):

- Gross revenue trends in recent years
- Profit trends
- Practice growth in real terms (bearing in mind the impact of inflation)
- Case volume
- The level and significance of each of the practice costs
- Liquidity
- Cash flow
- Debtor level
- Stock turnover
- Gearing

Now you have some indication of where you are in financial terms. You will need to decide what specific financial objectives to set over the period of the plan, calculate the level of income you will need to generate, and estimate the costs of achieving that income.

Possibly you have assumed that practice profits are largely the result of influences beyond your control. Maybe you take the view that the practice deals with all the clinical work that presents itself but that its financial performance must look after itself. You note with some interest at your financial year end what costs you incurred. You express satisfaction or dismay at the profit level you achieved.

Take Control

We urge you to set your financial strategy in motion and take control of what happens in the practice.

STEP 1: Decide now what profit figure you intend to achieve each year in your two-year strategy. Be bold and specific. Write it down.

STEP 2: Examine the practice costs last year. Rethink every single cost item. Identify the property, equipment and personnel resources you are likely to need over the period. Isolate the fixed and variable costs of those resources in financial terms or as a proportion of practice turnover.

STEP 3: Calculate what level of revenue the practice will need to generate in order to finance those costs and achieve a surplus, the profit level you have already determined. Remember that practice revenue is simply a function of case volume and the value of the average transaction. This gives you a number of possible options for increasing turnover and improving the quality of service to clients.

You could for example:

- INCREASE case volume by implementing a variety of clinical or marketing policies for growth.
- INCREASE the fee for each service item to position your practice in the demographic marketplace.
- INCREASE charges for products sold, dispensed or utilised in providing those services.
- INCREASE the services rendered or products sold during each transaction.

Each of the last three measures will result in an increased average transaction value. The practice must monitor case volume and average transaction value on a regular basis. The simplest approach is to regard each chargeable invoice as one unit of volume.

An important part of your financial plan is to define clearly how you intend to generate the target income level. What trends you are able to anticipate for case volume, fees and average transaction values.

Financial Projections

Your strategic financial plan should include projected profit and loss statements for each of the next two years and a detailed monthly cash flow budget for the first year.

No matter how carefully you plan, the projections can only give a broad indication of what you expect to happen in the future. Give an indication in your plan of the best possible scenario, the worst, and your estimate of the likeliest outcome.

Whenever possible, put your financial projections on a computer spreadsheet. Changes are instantaneously accommodated. Throughout the year, you will be updating and tinkering with your assumptions and within seconds will be able to consider the anticipated outcome they will create.

Cash Flow Statement

A major benefit of preparing cash flow statements regularly is to keep the bank manager appraised of progress. Bank managers are generally positive and helpful but they don't like unpleasant surprises. Work on the basis of keeping one step ahead. Cash flow forecasting will enable you to notify the bank two or three months ahead if you anticipate significant changes in your overdraft or other requirements. Oversights here or inadequate financial planning can prove to be embarrassing and expensive. Younger practices with less working capital are especially vulnerable.

The statement should incorporate the assumptions used to identify the various cost items as well as the positive steps which could be taken to ensure revenue targets are achieved. The financial plan will include significant anticipated capital expenditures over the period with an outline timetable, the method of payment, likely costs and an indication of the additional income expected from the investment. Finally, include a review of the funding of the practice and incorporate a brief indication of likely balance sheet values for each of the two years ahead.

The Marketing Plan

Your business plan will need to incorporate a marketing strategy. Marketing as an important management role is dealt with in detail in Chapter 4 but your written plan will certainly need to include a statement about the market and some answers to the following questions:

- What is happening in the outside world to affect the practice? (Political, economic, environmental, social and technological trends all have an influence, positive or adverse, on your practice plan.)
- What local situations may affect business?
- What is happening to the market for veterinary services in the catchment area for your practice?
- Who are your competitors and what other sources of animal health advice and products are available for your clients or potential clients?
- What are your competitors doing better or worse than you?
- What is special about your practice?
- What is your practice image and how do you want to be perceived?
- Who are your clients?
- Where do they reside?
- What animals do they own and what services do these patients require?
- What are your clients willing to pay?
- Are you satisfying their existing needs or does the system inhibit you and your staff from satisfying those needs?
- Are you innovative enough to anticipate client needs in the future?
- How do you know what your clients need now or may need in the future? Have you asked them?

Simply satisfying clients is not enough. You have to satisfy their needs profitably. Sustainable profit in veterinary practice comes from clients who boast about your practice attributes and come back regularly bringing friends with them.

The traditional veterinary approach has been to build long-term relationships with clients. Do you ask satisfied clients regularly for referrals and thank them when they do? The purpose of a veterinary practice is to create and keep clients. Offer services that clients want and value. Clients must perceive these services as better than those offered by colleagues at competitive prices.

The marketing-oriented veterinarian recognises that successful practice is primarily a client-satisfying service rather than a location for practising veterinary medicine. Meet and exceed client expectations.

Overworked or Underworked?

What about your needs as far as the market is concerned?

- Are you overworked?
- Are there too many clients?
- Is there a danger that pressure of work could result in a declining standard of service?
- Do you need more employees?
- Have you thought about investing some time and resources into a continuing professional development programme to help you to put your professional life into perspective?
- Do you need a holiday?
- Is your increasing involvement in other interests outside practice (e.g. veterinary politics, local politics, charitable or voluntary organisations or other business ventures) restricting the time you are able to devote to your practice or are your premises, equipment and staff working below capacity?
- Could you serve more clients to ensure that all your facilities are utilised in a cost-effective manner and that every case makes a significant contribution to your fixed costs?

If your problem is overwork, you may consider a number of options. Perhaps you should restrict the range of services you offer or the number of your clients. Retain only those that satisfy your own professional wishes or which are the most cost-effective. You can be more financially and professionally successful with a select client base. When necessary have the courage to deal with your headaches by counselling difficult clients to move to neighbouring colleagues!

If you need more clients or if your practice strategy depends on growth you will want to consider increasing practice revenue and promoting practice services offered. A number of choices for generating additional work exist. The traditional marketing matrix approach incorporates four options: You may promote existing services to existing clients, existing services to new clients, new services to existing clients, or new services to new clients.

Remember that your existing client database, on computer or card, is your most valuable marketing asset. The most cost-effective marketing investment you can make is to ensure that your current clients are fully aware of the wide range of services your practice can offer now and which of them are appropriate for their animals. You may not be comfortable with the concept of 'selling your services' but you will surely want to ensure that every client is offered the best possible professional advice. Given the opportunity to consider and to accept that advice, clients may respond far more positively than you may anticipate.

Marketing is simply an understanding of the marketplace in which your practice exists; the needs, spoken or unspoken, of your clients and potential clients, and the development and provision of the products or services they require, if they can be offered ethically and profitably.

The People Plan

Practice success depends absolutely on the knowledge, skills, enthusiasm, hard work, dedication and commitment of every single individual who works in the practice. You, your partners and your staff are all stakeholders in the success of the business. Your business plan must include some answers to the following people questions.

- Who are the people in the practice: you, your partners and all your staff?
- What is their role, who does what, how do you divide their tasks and responsibilities?
- What qualifications and skills do they have?
- What are your present manpower strengths and weaknesses? Draw up a list.
- What tasks are you doing well?
- What tasks could you do better?
- What tasks are you failing to do at all and why? Is it a shortage of skills or of manpower?
- What is missing and how can you obtain them (staff or skills)? Remember it might be cheaper to train your existing staff than to recruit or replace them.

Your Ability to Lead and Manage

When you consider practice personnel strengths and weaknesses, don't forget that one of the key features to judge is your ability and that of your colleagues to carry out the wide range of management roles which will be required.

Ask your partner, professional or personal, to score your ability against the following skills. They are offered as a suggested list of attributes and you might find it useful to use them to identify specific characteristics which are worth looking for in prospective professional colleagues.

How Do You Score?

How do you and your colleagues, score on a scale of 1 to 10 for each attribute?

- Leadership
- Judgement
- Entrepreneurial flair
- Psychological stamina
- Goal identification
- Decision making
- Delegation
- Whim resistance
- Dependability
- Application

They haven't been listed in any particular order of importance except for 'leadership' at the top of the list. Leadership is the characteristic of the individual with the dream, the vision for the future and the charisma which can fire the imagination of those who follow to share that vision.

Leadership is much more than being the boss. It's about a sense of direction and knowing the next step. Leadership is not sufficient alone.

Many leaders are not necessarily good at administration or managing resources. What leaders are good at is inspiring others — managers may be appointed, bosses may appoint themselves but a hospital director is never really a leader until accepted by those he leads. The best veterinary practice principals are the leaders. They have identified their vision, established a practice style, expect performance, formulate ideas and plans and then implement them.

Summary

A practice business plan must incorporate three major sections besides an overall strategic mission statement. A financial plan, a marketing plan and a personnel plan are the kernels of a seed plan. The following chapters deal with each of them in some detail.

Why not take the first step now. Fix a time and date in your diary NOW. Tell your colleagues in the practice that you are taking the lead and preparing a business plan for the practice. Everyone will need to be involved and fully support the endeavour.

DO IT NOW! — DO IT NOW WITH A PLAN!

4

Veterinary Marketing

The Veterinary Marketplace

Marketing has been described as the task of examining the whole business enterprise from the consumer's point of view. Pose and answer questions such as:

- What business am I in?
- Who are my clients?
- Where do they come from?
- What do they want, or not want?
- Can the business provide what is required and at what price?

The objective is to highlight the importance for every practice principal of giving some thought to the marketplace in which the practice operates. They should identify what is happening to that market and the likely impact of market changes on the range, quality and price of the services provided. No business plan is complete unless it incorporates some reference to marketing.

Market Trends

Life implies change. Nothing stays static for very long. Practising veterinary surgeons operate in a dynamic marketplace and need to recognise the significance of worldwide changes and trends. Changes in the local environment must also be considered and steps taken to modify and extend the services offered as a result of those trends.

Someone once said, 'If you do what you've always done, you'll get what you've always got!'. Consumers are changing so rapidly that practices who 'do what they've always done' may no longer 'get what they've always got'. The world changes. The style and quality of service providing a very good living a few years back may not now fit the bill.

Veterinary clients are typical consumers, increasingly concerned about quality, cost, service,

reliability and convenience. Some may well switch their loyalties to another veterinary practice in the vicinity if they perceive that the competing practice scores better in those attributes. Professional experience or skills may be very similar, but clients are also attracted by their perception of a professional's sensitivity to their needs and those of their animals.

Look closer at how consumers are changing. No two people are quite the same. Identify some general trends which may affect clients in the marketplace. Consumers are just people. People today are now better off, more discerning, more widely travelled, more demanding, better educated and less tolerant. They want and expect their wishes to be satisfied immediately, not tomorrow. The emphasis today is to seek to maintain health. Consumers seek fast, high-tech, modern services, but they also want to do their bit for the environment.

They are attracted by 'one stop shopping'. Some are primarily concerned with quality and not too concerned about cost. Some are extremely cost conscious and still want quality, but all seek value for money.

A trend is developing away from 'the middle ground'. Consumers for a wide range of goods and services are positively moving 'up-market' or 'down-market'. Suppliers of goods and services have traditionally tried to please all the people all the time but may now find themselves increasingly losing out.

Consensus within the profession is that veterinary practices undercharge. Fees are far too low. Veterinarians are 'frightened by large invoices'. If this is so, then raising fees and choosing to go up-market, will ensure the highest professional standards, care and service matching fee increases. If all practices follow the trend upwards, the needs of the large, cost conscious section of the market at the bottom end may not be satisfied. In a free market economy someone will seek to satisfy that market. The practising arm of the profession may then have to cope with the problems of low-cost neutering and vaccination clinics and other animal health services.

In spite of the economic recession of the last two or three years, people today have much more disposable income than they have ever had. They have more credit cards to buy more freezers, videos, microwave ovens, long haul holidays, computer games and private health insurance. Purchasing has accelerated at a rate higher than imagined a few years back.

Consumers with money are getting older — the so called greying trend. A significant increase in the number of single-parent families has also evolved. Cynics welcome the increase in the numbers of marriages ending in divorce. A couple who own a pet and divorce, may well end up as 'two good clients' with 'two good veterinary patients'. A trend continues towards smaller families. Pets continue to be surrogate children for some couples. An increasing recognition of the importance of the human/animal bond has benefitted veterinary medicine.

The market today is a buyer's market. Clients have less free time and seek convenience goods and services. As special, unique individuals, they are attracted much less by the mass provision of goods or services.

The Need to Compete

Competition in the animal health and welfare market becomes keener all the time. Veterinary surgeons find it difficult to recognise that they are in competition. It might be unethical to do or say anything which implies that their practice is in any way superior to any other or that the service they are able to offer is better.

The inescapable truth is that the interests of owners and their animals are best served in a marketplace where there are a number of service providers. No single practice is able to satisfy the requirements of all the people all the time. Some like the hustle and bustle of a large busy practice with the perceived benefits of a well equipped and efficient large enterprise. A number of veterinary

surgeons and lay staff are employed to provide a wide range of services. Some clients are much happier dealing with a single veterinary surgeon in a small personal practice environment.

Practitioners have traditionally been advised that the best possible place to set up a new practice is almost next door to a thriving large veterinary hospital. Why? — because the new practice would attract all those clients who currently go to the large hospital but who are fed up with high fees, never seeing the same veterinarian twice, the left hand not knowing what the right is doing, and so on.

All veterinary practices are in a competitive business. They compete for a share of their clients' disposable income. Money which, if it is not spent on their animals, might be spent on the home, the garden, holidays, clothes or drink.

By and large, veterinary clients are faithful to the practice where they have received high standards of service over many years. But things change. The veterinarians in the practice change, the staff change, the nature of the competition changes and the financial circumstances and perceived needs of the client or patient, may also change.

A major component of the marketing plan must be to promote the practice as one which is special and which has some unique characteristics. A practice which is perceived to be the same as all the rest, has no image at all. The public cannot make a reliable, informed choice based on competence. Generally clients perceive that all veterinarians are competent professionals.

Effective professional competition then depends on enhanced levels of quality and service. Specialty or other non-traditional services are offered to clients which may be unique to the marketplace. Competition must be welcomed! When the veterinary marketplace is allowed to function unhindered, everybody is a winner - clients and practitioners. The only losers are those who provide an inadequate level of services. Professional ability must always be honoured. What has been good enough in the past will not continue to be good enough in the future.

In practical terms, how can you compete with all the other successful practices in your neighbourhood?

- Carry out an audit of all the practices in the locality
- Seek the help of a member of your staff, a friend or relative or better still, have a word with one of your oldest and most faithful clients. Ask them to examine other practice premises critically.
- How do your competitors respond to telephone calls? What reputation do they have in the locality and how do they compare with what you offer?
- What are other practices doing very much better than you are?
- What are you doing better than them?
- What lessons can you learn?
- How can your practice build on its strengths or take effective action to correct some of its shortcomings?

Increasingly successful veterinary practices will be those in which the practice owner or principal is obsessed by total quality management. Continue to thirst for professional and business knowledge, maintain the highest possible professional and ethical standards, and ensure that every member of the staff understands and shares those values.

Clients seek value for money. They are concerned with cost but price is only one of those factors which animal owners take into account in choosing their veterinary adviser. Veterinarians should compete on quality of service, not price. If some clients complain about fees, concentrate on improving the value of the service provided.

What are the lessons to be learned? What are the implications for the practising veterinary surgeon?

Animal owners seek advice on products and services, and about the health and welfare of their pets. Their first impulse is not necessarily or automatically to seek such advice from their local veterinary practice. There are plenty of other sources of information: pet shops, animal health merchants, supermarkets, pharmacists, breeders, boarding kennels, animal behaviourists and a host of others.

Veterinarians have to strike a very careful balance between idealism and capitalism. Professional obligations and a code of ethics rightly emphasise the interests of the patient as being paramount.

Alternatively, global competition establishes the necessity of being consumer-, rather than service-oriented. These obligations are not mutually incompatible. The over-riding philosophy must be to provide the very best level of professional service. It would be irresponsible not to ensure that our clients are fully aware of what is available, that they are offered the best and that they are then allowed to make up their own minds to choose the best.

The Marketing Plan

Write down what you want. Do you need more clients or are you already overworked, underpaid and not in a position to satisfy your existing clients let alone seek new ones? How long and how hard do you want to work? How important is your leisure? Either way you urgently need a marketing plan.

Having a positive marketing plan is very definitely not about turning veterinary surgeons into slick salesmen. That would be bad ethics and very bad for business. Selling is concerned with the interests of the vendor. Marketing is much more concerned with benefits for the client. Marketing embraces the educational relationship between clinician and client in the best interests of the patient.

Practice Image

Look at your own organisation critically to eliminate anything, however small, which might damage the perception of the practice in the eyes of your clients or other animal owners in the vicinity. Be sensitive to the special needs of children, the elderly, the infirm, and the disabled.

In marketing terms, perception is reality. Client retention may be more important than client acquisition. It is probably true that only a small proportion of clients who believe that they have cause for complaint, actually complain. The problem is that whilst those few of your clients who are dissatisfied may not complain to you, they will probably air their grievances with other people. Your other clients or potential clients may hear all about the bad news about your practice before you do.

The lesson is to ensure that any clients who have cause for complaint, however trivial, are encouraged to let you or your staff members know. Most complaints result from failed expectations. Your front-line non-professional staff play an invaluable communication role in preventing and dealing with many of the problems which might arise.

Albrecht and Zemke refer to the metaphor of the 'moment of truth' as a powerful idea for helping people in service industries and professions. Daily, we all make personal, subjective, subconscious judgments about the shops we visit, the services we seek, and the contacts we make. When we visit a restaurant, we are affected by the external appearance, the welcome we get from the staff, the smell of the cuisine being prepared, the temperature and the appearance of the interior and the service we receive, all affect our perception of value. The quality and appearance of the food and the price we pay are significant factors but are not of overwhelming importance in moulding our opinion. Each of these judgments helps us build an overall impression of the business. In turn, all of these factors will influence our decision to go back or to stay away.

So it is with veterinary practice. Clients may visit a practice once and never return. In the United States it is reported that 38% of new clients never come back. Why? Just think how many moments of truth could influence a new client visiting your practice for the first time. You only have one opportunity for a first impression.

- Is the practice easy to find?
- Can the client park easily?
- Is the car park clean and tidy?
- On opening the front door, is there any unpleasant smell?
- Does the receptionist make eye contact immediately, even if she is busy?
- Is a client's presence acknowledged?
- Is the client enthusiastically welcomed, spoken to, assisted?

A client in a practice for maybe three minutes, who hasn't even seen the veterinarian yet, has already made subconscious but valid judgements which play an important part in developing their future attitude to the practice.

Know Your Market

Write down what you know about the market in your area.

- Who are your clients?
- What sort of people are they?
- What animals do they own?
- What services do they require?
- Where do they come from?
- How do they get to your practice?
- How often do they come to your practice?
- How much do they spend at your practice each year?

If you don't know the answers perhaps you should work with your front-line reception and nursing staff to find out. What specifically do your clients need — comfort, security, care, someone to listen, consistency, reliability, trust, no negatives (no smells, no waits, no weeds)? What benefits are they buying? Pet owners don't have an overwhelming desire to buy a vaccination course for their young puppy. It involves time, they have to phone to make an appointment, take an unwilling animal to be examined and injected and spend money! What they do want to buy is peace of mind, a healthy pet, an active happy companion and the self esteem that they are doing the right thing. Are these the benefits that you are promoting?

External Influences

What national or international issues are affecting your clients? Veterinary practices aren't immune from the social, political and economic issues that affect any other business. Which of these issues is likely to affect your veterinary business? They will all affect your practice to some extent but some (e.g. agricultural policies in the EC, the world recession, zoonoses, animal welfare and environmental issues) will probably have a greater impact than some others.

Market Share

Can you estimate how many farms, stables, households or people there are in the catchment area for your practice?

- How many horses, cattle, sheep, pigs, hens, dogs, cats or exotic animals are owned in the area?
- What proportion of the whole are 'your clients'?
- If your strategic plans succeed what share of the market will you need?
- Identify all the other veterinary practices, welfare societies and other providers of animal health services and advice in the area. Write down what you know about them.
- How many veterinarians do they employ?
- What image do they have?
- What services do they provide?
- Which are better than yours?
- What does your practice do better than the others?
- How many full time 'veterinarian equivalents' are busy in your market?
- What is the relationship between the number of veterinarians and the population of people, pets, horses or farm animals in the area?
- Would you judge that the area is blessed with an over-abundance of veterinarians?
- What are the opportunities for growth?
- Do you try and satisfy all the people all the time?
- Do you succeed?

If you have too many clients maybe you should concentrate your efforts on those who seek, appreciate and are happy to pay for the style of service you want to provide. Gently ease out the rest. If you want to grow, maybe you should match the service you offer, specifically to the segment of the animal-owning market that you wish to encourage. Do you want to be 'all things to all men' or should you be selective? Should you seek a unique niche market? Write down your conclusions.

The worth of a practice can actually increase by abandoning a particular segment of activity. A predominantly small animal mixed practice may not have a sufficient large animal volume to justify pursuit of that market. In fact, the large animal segment may be generating losses subsidised by the small animal division. A marketing plan may recognise this accounting reality. Paring down your market focus may improve both profit margin percentage and amount. Some practice owners however, may recognise the economic reality of the situation but wish to continue to serve the unprofitable market segment because they enjoy it.

Practice Services

Now turn your mind to the various services you currently offer.

- Which services do you find boring, uninteresting or a nuisance?
- What skills and services, current or potential do you find exciting, thrilling or fascinating?
- What services have you identified that your clients would welcome but which you can't yet deliver?
- What investment would be required to fill in the gaps?
- Which of your services generate the most revenue?
- Which of them contribute the most to the bottom line?
- Do you know?
- Should you find out?
- How?

Which of your services are your 'cash cows'? — those services which provide the bread and butter, the bulk of your practice income? The important thing here is to maintain your standards, concentrate on quality, maintain your enthusiasm and concentrate on building committed clients for your practice.

Are there any services which you might regard as 'rising stars'? — those services which you think have considerable potential but which need some initial investment. Perhaps advice for behavioural problems, laboratory profiles, comprehensive dentistry, nutritional management of disease and maybe merchandising are good examples of veterinary 'rising stars' in your practice.

Are there any services which provided your bread and butter in the past but which appear now to be declining as a proportion of the whole? Marketers call these 'dead dogs' — perhaps an unfortunate phrase under the circumstances. Are there any changes on the horizon which are likely to shatter the status quo? It wouldn't be at all surprising.

Summarise your proposals for promoting or advertising the practice during the next year or so. Should you allocate part of your budget for that purpose? How much do you think would be appropriate? How much did you spend last year on advertising the practice in Yellow Pages, other directories, local newspapers or direct mail to your clients with newsletters, booster reminder letters and other material? What was the payback? Was it worthwhile? Many practices advertise in Yellow Pages. The Yellow Pages investment with multi-colour block advertisement space when available, is expensive but, dependent upon the demographic area, the expense may be justified. Transient client areas benefit from Yellow Pages emphasis. Practices with aggressive colleagues who advertise boldly may force other practices to respond in kind. Other practice areas with stable long term residents and sensible colleagues may not have the need to use commercial telephone listings. Practitioners should regard their investment in promoting their services to existing clients as equally as important as searching for new clients. Direct mail, client handouts, and other material provide a much better and more readily measurable financial return. Direct mailing clients with personalised letters is one of the most effective forms of advertising. The more you are able to target clients in particular areas, or clients owning animals in particular age groups or with particular problems, the more cost effective your advertising budget will be.

Remember, the best and the least expensive form of advertising is by word of mouth. Satisfied clients spread the word about the attributes of the best practice in the area — your practice. Thank them for their efforts on your behalf and provide them with plenty of practice brochures to distribute amongst their animal owning acquaintances.

Consider your existing vaccination booster reminder system. Veterinarians generally recognise the importance of booster vaccination reminders to generate additional revenue. Many practices are unable to calculate their impact on profits or the response which is achieved to primary and follow-up booster vaccination reminders. What system to use? — postcards, personalised letters or telephone? What response rate is achieved now? How many patients are up to date with their immunisation programme? Is it at least 65%? Do you know? Should you find out? How?

Veterinarians may not be aware of the number of animals under their care that are not up to date with their vaccine programme. Positive steps must be taken to inform clients. Is a practitioner failing his ethical responsibilities if he does not ensure that clients who own animals under his care are positively and regularly informed of the need to maintain a vaccination programme? Perhaps so — and its not very good for business!

The next stage of your marketing plan is to set some specific practice marketing policies and targets. Consider:

- Your practice policies on fees. What principles are used to establish them?
- What precisely are your practice's 'cash cows', 'rising stars' and 'dead dogs'?
- What positive steps are needed to understand the market in which the practice operates?
- What positive projections are you prepared to make and over what period will they operate?
- What volume targets need to be set for each range of service?
- What about specific services? How many ECGs, dentals, laboratory profiles, etc. do you intend to carry out during the next twelve months?
- Plans cannot be achieved alone. Discuss them with your colleagues and your staff. Solicit the staff's help to achieve practice targets. If set by everyone in the practice, practice targets have a higher probability of being hit.

A Strategy for Growth

Develop an agreed written practice protocol. Documentation ensures that the approach to clinical cases by all the veterinary surgeons in the practice is similar and that the practice policy in respect of recalls, re-examinations, referrals, laboratory workups and other diagnostic tools is carried out by all the staff involved.

Always tell the client exactly how it is. Veterinarians should make clinical judgements in the best interests of the patient and advise the client accordingly. Give the client time to make a decision to accept your advice for better veterinary medicine, management or surgery. For example, if your professional judgement is that all animals over a certain age should be subject to some laboratory investigation prior to anaesthesia, then say so! Recommend the test to your client. If the answer is no — you might refuse to carry out the procedure or ask your client to sign a consent form declining your professional recommendation. You may however, feel that even a client's waiver may not satisfy your professional responsibility. You then have a choice either to refuse to perform the surgery or carry out the profile at no charge. An ethic for professional excellence may on occasions overcome economic prudence.

Set specific marketing objectives for the practice. Targets should be realistic, certainly not too easy but challengingly achievable. Making 'sales' targets is very much a team effort. Goals are often tougher and more likely to be reached if those who have to do the work are also involved in setting the targets.

Jot down your thoughts about targets for the practice such as;

- increase the number of ECG reports by 15% within three months,
- promote dental services in cats and increase case volume by 20% by June 1st,
- improve the response to vaccine booster recalls from 60% to 70% by the end of the year.

The possible list is endless. Don't try to do too much too soon. Choose a few, get the staff positively involved, consider implementing a performance related pay system and monitor the results.

A Strategy for Fees

Concentrate on value not price. Never apologise for your fee structure (and make sure your staff don't either). Teach staff that the approach always should be 'we can provide this service for as little as....' The level of fees is irrelevant — £50, $100 or ECU200 if the value of the service you offer is perceived by your clients as £55, $120 or ECU250!!!

A practice's professional staff is sensitive about fees. Donald Dooley believes that veterinarians are born with a fear of large numbers. They quickly develop a subconscious maximum fee in their minds. You should aim to establish a system which completely separates the veterinarians on a day to day basis from any responsibility for deciding the fees to be charged for individual clients. Veterinarians approach fee setting with a degree of fear and trembling that clients will love them less if the fees are too high. But times are changing. We recognise that it is hard to put a charge on the value of your own expertise when newly graduated but, in some practices it is the young veterinarians who set the pace and have a hard task to persuade the practice owners to follow their lead to charge at a realistic level.

A computer system can help transfer that fear. A clinician can team up with his clients versus the machine, 'Look how much the computer has charged us today (note the 'us') Mrs Smith. Still for that price you can be satisfied that Charlie is getting the best care'. However, be judicious in invoking the editorial 'we' or you may be convinced by a persuasive client to override the decision of the electronic brain!.

Bear in mind those few charges over which some animal owners 'shop around'. Price competitively for spays, castrations, and vaccinations whilst ensuring that you charge realistically for everything else. Don't ever get trapped by charging fees which are 'affordable'. Only your clients can decide what they can or choose to afford. It is all a question of priorities. Just offer the best, quote the price and let the client decide. Unless you charge a 'fair fee', you will soon be out of business. By giving services away, a veterinarian ensures the continued longevity of colleagues who will be able to generate a reasonable profit to feed their families and stay afloat. Charge too little and expect a short professional career. Professional burnout rarely afflicts the financially prudent practitioner.

Never try to hide the costs. Always give an estimate and pitch it higher than the total fee you expect. The client will be delighted with a satisfactory outcome to the problem and a fee significantly less than expected. Client dissatisfaction always arises when expectations are higher that performance. Make sure that seldom happens in your practice.

Charge for everything you do. How much extra do you charge when you empty the patients anal sacs during a routine consultation? or instil fluorescein in its eye? — nothing! — don't you — then why not? But don't go overboard. Charging is an art form, not a science. Use your common sense. Be firm but be flexible when it is necessary. Empower your staff also to be flexible on occasions — but ensure that they are prepared to defend their decisions if and when you challenge them.

Don't ever get left behind. Keep up with and ahead of inflation and every time you increase your fees review the quality of the service you offer. Try to identify your clients needs and do better — much better! Become a fanatic for quality and charge accordingly.

Make a note every time a client complains to you or your staff about your fees. Record the complaint on the patient record card and on your monthly staff agenda to discuss the comment. Compare notes with other practice members to identify patterns of dissatisfaction.

Don't forget to date your price lists and see if the complaints go up when the fees do. Try to decide what is about right. If you never get a complaint about the price of your services you should be ashamed — they must be far too low. A rate of 5% complaining and 2% leaving is probably about right.

What about practice image? Pretend an executive couple were planning to move into your town. They own a couple of Irish Setters and three cats. Before deciding to purchase a property they are anxious to identify a good veterinary practice and spend the evening in a local motel or hostelry and talk 'dogs, cats and veterinarians'. What will they hear about your practice? Do you know? Do you

think they will hear what you would like them to hear? What would you like them to hear? Could you write down now in approximately 200 words or fewer, an outline sketch of the image and attributes of your practice? As a good exercise, stop reading and start writing.

Believe that the appearance of the practice and your staff and the way they communicate with clients is an important part of your required practice image. Telephone your own practice from time to time (disguise your voice if need be) and see how you are treated. Try this with other practices too. Do you think that dress and proper grooming are important? Do you think that veterinarians should look like veterinarians, smart and professional or do you think that a shirt and tie and clean shoes are a sign of impending senility? If you do think that such values are important say so and don't tolerate anything less. Share your thoughts with your staff. Let them know about your vision of the practice image and listen to what they say.

Focus on Quality

If quality is a component part of your practice image, develop an obsession with quality in everything you do. Remember the acronym TREAT;

TANGIBLE RESOURCES; Consider the condition and the appearance of your premises and your professional, office and other equipment, fixtures and fittings. Do they help to reinforce the image that you are seeking for quality? If not, what should you do about it?

RESPONSIVENESS; Does your practice respond quickly to the needs of your clients. Is your practice response willing, enthusiastic, supportive and helpful?

EMPATHY; Are the people in your practice; you, your colleagues and all your staff members perceived as warm, sympathetic, caring and prepared to offer time and individual attention?

ASSURANCE; Can your clients be assured of the skills, service, expertise, courtesy, trust and confidence which they will receive from your practice today and every day?

TOTAL RELIABILITY; Does your practice carry out its responsibilities, provide the services offered and deliver what was promised to all your clients, always?

What would be the worst thing to hear about your practice other than that you cared more about making money than looking after animals? If the practice was perceived to be the same as every other practice in the town, it would be a pathetic commentary. Make sure that your practice is unique, special and manifest that quality to others so that they know what it is that makes it so much better and so different from all the others.

Identify all the ways that your practice is different. Do you or your staff members have special or unique professional skills or knowledge? Does your practice run extended consulting hours, early mornings or late evenings, with or without a fee premium? Can you provide an ambulance service? Consider a monthly newsletter targeted to a specific group of clients and with detailed information specifically for that target group, (e.g. Doberman owners, the owners of all your obese canine patients, clients with animals over seven years of age, clients owning dogs with congestive heart failure). The possibilities are endless. You will certainly get a better response than to a general newsy mailing. Can your practice offer specific laboratory services or encourage preventive medicine? Do you run 'well animal' clinics, geriatric clinics, or obesity clinics? The important point then is to monitor the percentage of invoices with a component relating to these services, to set targets and to monitor the results.

The Marketing Matrix

Marketing professionals talk about the marketing matrix. The matrix is simply a reminder that existing services can be offered to existing or potential clients. A practice can also develop and provide new services for existing clients or to potential clients.

Many practices spend a great deal of time and effort to work out ways of developing and promoting new services and seeking new clients. A little thought would make them realise that a more cost effective investment is to spend a limited marketing budget to ensure that existing clients are aware of the wide range of services

which is already available. Ensure too, that whenever appropriate they are making use of them.

Some services will not be appropriate for certain client's animals — but many will. Can you be sure, for example, that all of your small animal clients owning dogs or cats older than seven years, are aware of the particular knowledge, expertise and resources that you have invested in providing a geriatric monitoring service in the practice? Have you offered detailed monitoring of health problems?

You or your colleagues may already have a specialist interest in a particular sphere of professional knowledge. You may be planning a personal programme of continuing professional development. Remember that the skill you acquire will have a value. It may enable your practice to develop a unique service in your locality.

Salesmen talk about a USP — a unique selling point. It may be that your expertise with reptiles, insects, geriatric care, dentistry, exotic pets, equine fertility or any one of hundreds of other examples may be the USP which your practice can offer. The world has been in recession and times have been difficult for all businesses. Precisely, when competition is tough, professional practices, like all businesses, need to identify and develop a USP or a marketing niche in which they can excell.

Once determined, a specific new service development for the practice will be an important component of your overall marketing plan. Precisely who will be providing the service, what category of patients are to be targeted and how will you indicate to clients what is on offer? You will need to prepare a detailed clinical protocol to ensure that all the staff members are aware of the details and the procedures to be followed.

- How will you make a clinical evaluation and a diagnosis?
- What dietary, management, medical or surgical approach will you take?
- What additional equipment, staff skills, stock items or other materials will be required?
- What paperwork will need to be planned?
- What fees will you charge?

- How will you or your staff monitor the project, the numbers involved, the revenue generated and the additional costs incurred
- How and when will you be in a position to judge the outcome?

Consider too, how the service will be delivered. If it depends on the skill of one veterinarian you should consider providing a back-up to ensure that client expectations, which you have worked so hard to generate, are not disappointed.

Don't forget the positive marketing advantage of employing keen, enthusiastic veterinarians brimming with knowledge. Nurture them, encourage them, support them and help them to become better than you. The practice benefits two ways. The expertise brought to your practice can be used to develop and improve the level of professional expertise. That makes the practice special. In turn, experienced veterinarians in practice can pass on all those ideas which have been found so helpful in locking clients into their practice. Simple things like;

- using the client's and patient's name and talking to them both,
- introducing your staff by name to your clients,
    Dennis McCurnin suggests — 'always do something, say something, show something, give something and compliment the client and the patient',
- Listen to what the client says. Listening is an active pursuit, it requires concentrating on what is said and what really is of concern to the client.
- Involve your client in what you are doing and encourage a 'team approach' to solving the problem.

Maximise the value of staff meetings. They can be of benefit in a negative way, by providing an opportunity of airing, discussing and resolving small problems before they become too large and damaging. Meetings can also be invaluable in a positive way to encourage every member of the enterprise to become involved proactively. Help staff to 'own' the business plan for the practice and to make it clear that you believe that their special knowledge, experience and skills will be crucial if the plan is to be achieved. Be positive. Ask them; What are we doing right? How could we do this job better? Don't forget to listen to what they have to say.

Merchandising

Most veterinary practices dispense a range of medicines, dressings and other products to enable them to treat animals as out-patients under the direction of the consulting veterinarian. Many practices also sell a range of products to clients because of the need to provide a comprehensive service. They want to encourage animal owners to visit the practice to purchase food or other 'over-the-counter' products or to collect dispensed items even if there is no need to seek the individual advice of a veterinarian on that occasion. They work on the basis (rightly in our view) that regular clients, clients who are satisfied by the service they receive frequently, will be amongst the 20% who generate 80% of the practice revenue.

Some veterinarians are less comfortable about merchandising in practice and follow the pattern of traditional medical hospitals which are not generally involved in selling health products. Others take the view that the veterinary profession has copied the human hospital model too closely and that animal owners seek an all embracing 'cradle to grave' service for their animals.

Some believe that it is sensible and responsible to sell any product which will assist clients in solving an animal related problem. Others would judge it unwise to seek to compete by selling products available from local pet shops and other retail outlets.

The important point to make is that the matter should be debated and discussed within the practice. The views of clients and staff, as well as the people who might be involved in the policy should be taken into account before a decision is made.

No two veterinary practices are alike. Likewise, no two veterinarians will have the same viewpoint. Many believe that merchandising is acceptable if the products are chosen on the basis of professional judgment as well as on the contribution they make to profits.

When deciding to sell a range of animal care products in addition to specific pharmaceutical and essential stock items be sure to do the job properly. Consider merchandising as a specific profit centre project. Prepare a plan. Consider ethical and legal questions as appropriate in your country. Finally, identify the costs of shelving and other display units and any possible additional staffing and training costs.

Professional merchandising can enhance the reputation of a veterinary practice. If designed as an additional service, clients are encouraged to visit the practice more frequently. Appropriate products must be displayed properly in open shelves. Veterinarians and support staff must promote their value and their use positively and, as for any service, you must establish a proper accounting and recording system to ensure that the project makes a significant contribution to fixed costs.

Don't underestimate the necessity for training support staff. They must be fully aware of the value, features, and benefits associated with every product on sale and under what circumstances the product should be used. Remember that your practice image depends on the way your reception staff handle enquiries about retail sales in your reception area or waiting room. The role of the receptionist or other staff member is not simply to 'make a sale'. They must also ensure that clients are confident in their decision to come to your practice, seek advice and purchase the products recommended.

Most practice managers or principals will ensure that a single member of the staff takes responsibility for managing the merchandising unit and ensuring that pilfering by clients, casual visitors, or even by staff members, is kept to a minimum. Merchandising will be successful only if the veterinarian believes it will enhance the practice image and is determined to take the necesssary steps to implement the policy properly.

References

Service America – doing business in the new economy, Karl Albrecht and Ron Zemke, Dow Jones – Irwin, 1985.

5

Winning and Keeping Clients

Marketing in Your Reception Area

External marketing may be described as a study of the marketplace in relation to locality, the establishment of ethical services designed to satisfy that market and the steps taken to spread the news in a catchment area served by the practice.

Existing clients are your most valuable practice asset. An even more important marketing initiative must be designed to ensure that they receive the support and services they require. The decision to stay with a particular practice must be constantly reinforced. This may be described as internal marketing.

The Practice Receptionist

The reception staff play a pivotal role in ensuring the success, or failure, of a practice. They must understand the importance of practice image. They will be a large part of it.

Ask them:

What is the image of this practice?

How do you know?

How could you find out?

Is it the image you think the practice should have?

What is the image of the other practices in the area?

Is it your role to be interested in such matters? (of course it is!)

Be prepared to discuss the questions and their answers. Remind the staff that the perception that animal owners in a locality have about your practice is real. It may or may not reflect the reality accurately, but their decision to come to a particular practice or to visit the veterinary hospital around the corner will depend on their perception of the reality.

Ask them what clients grumble about. In even the best practices clients will from time to time complain about the services, staff, or fees. Nine times out of ten it will be the reception staff at the receiving end of the grumbles. You have to talk to them to be aware of your client's complaints. If you dont, you may not realise that a steady stream of clients is moving to the practice down the road because they don't wish to subject themselves to the rudeness or negative attitude of a professional colleague. Communicate with the reception staff regularly. Listen to what they have to say. Find out what problems they can identify and ask them what steps they would take to resolve them. Perhaps the clincher question is 'would you honestly choose to bring your animal to this practice if you didn't work here?'

The Reception Role

If you were to ask your reception staff to write down a list of all the jobs they were expected to do in the practice, what would be included? They would probably include some or all of the following:

- Record appointments, house calls and operations.
- Find clinical cards when, or before, the client arrives.
- Greet clients on their arrival.
- Prepare a client/patient record card or computer entry.
- Record details into the computer.
- Have appropriate clinical and financial records available for the veterinarian before the consultation.

- Answer the telephone.
- Prepare dispensed items as required.
- Prepare invoices.
- Ensure that all the rooms are clean and odour free.
- Ensure that all disposable items and routine items of equipment are available.
- Keep client flow as smooth as possible.
- As in-patients are released:
  - deal with all the paper work first.
  - make new appointments as necessary.
  - prepare and check an invoice.
  - arrange for veterinarian/client discussions about patient progress.
  - receive payment, record and receipt.
- Before releasing the patient, ensure that:
  - the client has made arrangements for travel (taxi or car).
  - the patient is awake, fit, groomed and clean (check with nursing staff before release).
- Deal with distressed, bereaved clients who may faint or be hysterical, aggressive or drunk.
- Cope with unruly children.
- Discuss a number of sensitive issues such as carcase disposal.
- File radiographs, computer printouts, correspondence and laboratory reports.
- Office filing and typing.
- Banking.
- Payroll.
- Daily book-keeping tasks.
- Sales ledgers.
- Process clients' cards.
- Management Accounting (manual or computer based).
- Purchase ledger.
- Monitor delivery notes, invoices, statements.
- Petty Cash.
- Monthly Accounts.
- Office Cleaning.
- Miscellaneous duties.

Have you thought recently how busy your reception staff are? What would be the consequences if any tasks on the list were not dealt with promptly and accurately? But there is so much more they could accomplish if given the lead and the resources required.

Here are just a few ideas in which reception staff can play a crucial marketing role in adding to the success of the practice:

- Monitor the response to clinical reminders.
- Credit control policies.
- Stock control policies (discuss margins, turnover, and stock levels).
- Generate more income.
- Promote 'over-the-counter' sales.
- Provide dietary management advice.
- Promote animal health insurance.
- Provide obesity control advice.
- Control waste (where does most waste occur? Have the appropriate staff been notified?)

Reception staff are also in an ideal situation to carry out mini-surveys from time to time to collect and collate marketing information for management. They can identify where clients come from, how often and how much they spend. They can also identify what clients appreciate and do not appreciate about your practice, and what services they might want — but are not available.

There are a number of specific topics which come high on the list of subjects for which reception staff seek specific help. They include:

Collecting Fees

Veterinary reception staff are much more comfortable and confident in collecting payment from clients when they understand the need for the practice to be profitable. A grasp of the significance of the fixed practice costs (i.e. the costs incurred whether or not clients telephone or visit the practice for advice) enables them to appreciate the level of investment required to provide those services.

When clients inquire about practice fees, ensure that the reception staff concentrate on value rather than price. 'The procedure for spaying your cat involves a thorough pre-operative clinical examination, a general anaesthetic, surgical removal of the uterus and ovaries, post-surgical monitoring and suture removal'. Outline the considerable benefits for the patient and the owner and indicate that 'we can provide this service for as little as $... — Would you like to arrange an appointment?'

Discuss and establish a formal policy for payment and ensure that the policy is clear to your staff and to your clients. Post a notice summarising your fee policy in a prominent position in the reception area. Consumers today are more used to paying for services as and when they receive them. The precise words which your reception staff use as clients return to the reception desk after services are rendered are crucial. 'The invoice comes to a total of $... Mrs. Jones. That includes the consultation, two injections, the antibiotic tablets and the blood test. Will you be paying by cash or cheque?' The routine must include receiving payment, giving a receipt and scheduling a follow-up appointment. It is the responsibility of the reception staff to ensure that any previous account balances are included in the total requested.

It is extremely important that a business routine is established in which practice principals and their staff expect to be paid at the time the service is rendered and that clients are aware that payment is to be tendered at that time. The routine should also offer clients a choice, but only a choice of two options (e.g. Would you prefer to pay by cash or credit card?, Would you like an appointment on Wednesday morning or afternoon?, Would you prefer the standard pack or the economy size?).

Many practices find it beneficial for reception staff to ask clients whether the veterinarians advice and instructions were clear and whether they require any other products or services before leaving.

Insist that the staff never apologise for your fees. If a client is convinced that the fees charged are appropriate for the quality of service provided, then staff members must be similarly convinced. Finally, concentrate on value for money. If adjustments need to be made — DON'T reduce the price — DO improve the quality.

Complaints

A marketing strategy will need to include your practice response to client complaints. The need to complain is sometimes legitimate. However well managed a practice may be, it is inevitable that some things will go wrong. A client may complain about some aspect of the service received. Complaints may, or may not be justified, but they must always be listened to with courtesy, in private, and responded to accordingly.

The important decision to make is to what extent a practice should actively encourage clients to comment when things go wrong or to complain when they feel it is necessary. What is the objective of the exercise? If a practice is obsessed with providing quality service and its marketing philosophy is to be client-oriented, it will want to attempt to convert the unhappy client to a satisfied one. On this basis then, you will want to establish a system which encourages unhappy clients to complain and give the practice the opportunity of putting matters right.

The practices response to complaints is crucial. Consider a situation in which you felt aggrieved by the standard of service you had received from a local garage. How would you feel if the response you received suggested you were wrong, that the complaint was unjustified, and that 'the experts know best'. I don't know about you, but I would be extremely irritated. I may or may not pursue the matter, but I would be most unlikely to return to that garage again.

On the other hand how would you react if the proprietor listened carefully to what you had to say, acknowledged that he understood the reason for your complaint and agreed to try to find a way of putting matters right. The question of the validity of your complaint is probably less important than the opportunity you had of expressing your concerns. Your decision to complain was acknowledged and a sincere effort was being made to resolve the problem.

Market research suggests that 70% of clients stay with practices which make an effort to remedy complaints. Moreover, as many as 95% want to repeat business with a practice that can remedy a problem on the spot.

How can a practice owner or manager begin to establish a policy for dealing with complaints? Remember the following:

- **Clients who complain are dissatisfied**. It is in the practice's best interest for the veterinarian to be aware of that dissatisfaction. Only by understanding the complaint can an owner or manager attempt to put matters right and retain the client.

- **Give clients every possible opportunity to express their dissatisfaction by allowing them time and privacy to do so.** Accept that the complaint is justified, explain any misunderstandings and apologise if necessary. Try to put matters right. The client is always right to complain, if they feel a need to complain.

Remember that management is all about monitoring the outcome of decisions. Once a practice establishes a routine for dealing with complaints, it needs to keep a formal record of them. Monitor how many complaining clients have been converted to long-term loyal clients who make a positive contribution to your practice growth. Monitor too, how many of your clients may be described as 'professional complainers' and determine a policy to deal with them.

Euthanasia

Inexperienced reception staff sometimes find the whole question of euthanasia for companion animals a difficult one with which to cope. They may understand and support the moral and scientific arguments for the need to end the lives of some animals because of intractable pain and an inability to lead a dignified life, but it takes different communication skills to discuss the issue with, and help, a distressed client.

Talk to your reception staff about the issue of euthanasia. Try to discover if they have any concerns or difficulties regarding euthanasia for animals and respond honestly and openly to their questions. There are a few practical points which are extremely important and which the staff should be aware of;

- Remember the importance of signed consent forms for all surgical, anaesthetic and diagnostic procedures and particularly for euthanasia cases. Always use the term 'euthanasia.' The term 'put to sleep' and other similar wordings **can** and **have been** misunderstood.

- Never blame the client for making a wrong decision, contrary to professional opinion, in having their animal euthanised. Little can be gained by seeking to argue about the issue after the fact. It is far better to offer sympathy and suggest that 'you feel sure that under the circumstances the decision was the right one'.

- Finally, caution your reception staff about being insensitive without meaning to be. For example, it would be inappropriate for a staff member to say to a distressed client, 'don't be too upset — she was only a dog (cat, gerbil, rabbit, white mouse....) — you can always get another one !'

Grief

Reception, nursing staff, and veterinarians sometimes find it difficult and embarrassing to communicate with a client who is grief-stricken after losing a beloved pet. Grief is a normal and natural emotion and it is usually possible to identify and understand the stages through which distressed clients pass.

Disbelief. The initial response is one of disbelief. 'Topsy can't be dead, she is only four and you told me the operation was a routine one'.

Anger Towards Others. Disbelief is quickly followed by anger. Anger towards the veterinarian, the nursing staff or a member of the family. Nursing and reception staff must accept that anger, understand it and allow it to be dissipated. They should try to offer sympathy and indicate that they care.

Anger Towards Themselves. Clients sometimes direct their anger against themselves. They feel guilty — 'it was all my fault, if we hadn't decided to cross the road on the bend, just when the bus was .....' Anger is frequently followed by feelings of depression and in due course, grief is replaced by happy memories.

These can be extremely difficult emotions to cope with in a busy veterinary practice. Here are two tips which may help in assisting staff members to cope:

- Understand the clients' distress. Never make light of the loss. Accept and understand it. Say something like, 'I understand how you feel Mrs. Johnson, Flossy was a wonderful companion and you will never be able to find another quite like her'.

- Do everything possible to help the client remember the good times they enjoyed with their pet, concentrate on the loss and the sadness and not the anger or guilt which are destructive emotions.

Price Shoppers

From time to time animal owners telephone the practice to identify the price range of routine vaccinations, surgical or other procedures. They are entitled to make any inquiries they wish. Telephone inquirers will discover a great deal more about a practice than simply the answer to the specific fee questions they pose.

An important marketing decision that must be made is how to respond to such inquiries. How does the staff feel about 'telephone shoppers'? Are they regarded as a nuisance or has a positive approach been designed to convert as many of them as possible into loyal clients? A practice protocol should include:

- asking if they are contacting other sources.
- indicating how sensible they are to do so.
- provide answers to their questions.
- indicate the level of quality service they will receive from your practice.
- ask if they wish to make an appointment (if the response is negative or cautious, offer to send information).
- note the name, address and telephone number and the names and species of their animals and send the information today.
- follow-up with a telephone call — ask whether they have all the information they required — again offer an appointment.
- monitor how many such calls are received and how many the staff were able to 'convert'.

Winning Clients for Your Practice

If there is one single objective which summarises the purpose of a reception staff, it is winning and keeping clients for your practice. Here are a few additional tips which reception staff can use to enhance their pivotal role in marketing policies:

- Effective communication. Communication is a two way process. Listening is probably more important than talking. More client dissatisfaction results from poor communication than inadequate professional service or advice.
- W.Y.B.O.W.T.S. — Simply an acronym which asks 'Would You Be Overjoyed With This Service?'
- Keep Children Occupied. Remember that 'Every day is Christmas — For the children!'. Reception staff can help clients and veterinarians both by keeping children occupied and amused during the consultation. A number of practices have collected toys, books and crayons which are invaluable when the reception area seems to be full of children.
- Quality and Accuracy of Information. Emphasise that your practice will be judged on the quality and accuracy of the information provided by the reception staff. They must be sure of their facts. If they are not sure, they must find out by referring to something or someone. Suggest that they build up a practice manual to include all the common questions that clients ask — together with the answers. Remind them that whilst they think they may know some of the answers, new employees may not be so fortunate.
- The client is always right — he or she pays your salary.
- Never say or do anything to make a client feel small or ridiculous.
- Every client is 'number one' in your practice.
- Never discuss or steam-roller a client's worries or objections. Try to allay those worries clearly and carefully. If the reception staff cannot allay those worries, then the veterinarian should speak to them.

In the eyes of the client, the perfect veterinary reception staff member NEVER:

- Shows obvious fear of an animal.

- Panics.
- Shows annoyance.
- Swears.
- Leaves a telephoning client 'on hold' without ensuring that they are prepared to wait.
- Discharges an animal dirty or bloody.

In the eyes of the client, the perfect reception staff member is ALWAYS:

- Kind, patient, polite and smart.
- Efficient, competent, sympathetic and in charge.
- Tactful and understanding.
- Quietly efficient and business-like.
- Gentle.
- Confident.
- Trustworthy.
- Sincere.
- Helpful.

Veterinarians have to believe in their marketing plan. If the practice owner believes in quality then they will practice quality. Make sure everyone in the practice knows that nothing less than the highest possible standards will be tolerated. The consequence will be that veterinarians and staff will promote the good news about veterinary practice all day every day. Offer only the best option and allow your clients to accept that advice.

Veterinary practice is a great leveller — we have all had days when Murphy's law reigned supreme and when everything that could go wrong has gone wrong. But we have also had days when we felt that we were the greatest veterinarian, nurse, technician, administrator, receptionist or manager there has ever been.

There is no greater feeling of satisfaction at the end of a busy day with all its ups and downs to recognise that you have done a good job — the job you have been trained to do well.

Have you prepared your marketing plan well?

Awareness and Attitude Studies

The essential principles of marketing may be summarised as follows:

- Examining consumer attitudes to existing services and suppliers.
- Finding out what consumers want — not simply what they ask for, but what they would like to have if they were aware of the possible options available to them.
- Providing the goods or services they want if it can be done ethically, legally and profitably.

A number of veterinary practices have found it invaluable to commission market research projects in the catchment area of their practice. They are designed to investigate the attitude of their own clients and of other animal owners in the locality towards their own practice and other competitor practices.

We offer the following exercise simply as an example of the type of questionnaire and the range of questions which may be considered of value in developing a marketing strategy. This particular example was used in a study for a typical small animal practice in a largely urban environment and with a number of competing practices in the marketplace.

Veterinarians should seek local professional advice to determine the number of completed questionnaires which are necessary to ensure the statistical validity of the results for management purposes. The appropriate catchment area size, the number of locations and details of the questions which are appropriate for any particular practice or project objective must also be determined.

Market Research Survey
Objective

This research project has been designed to examine the attitudes and opinions of the users of veterinary practices in the catchment area of the XYZ Animal Hospital.

The survey will be conducted at six urban locations within a five mile radius of the XYZ Animal Hospital and will take the form of street interviews with pet animal owners. The interviewers will use a detailed questionnaire custom-designed for the XYZ Animal Hospital.

The questions have been designed to probe for attitudes which might be below the surface and yet influence decision making by pet animal owners and help explain the dynamics of the market.

Here is an example of a typical local market research questionnaire.

Questionnaire

We are carrying out a survey into attitudes and opinions towards veterinary services in this area. If you have a pet animal in your household, would you be willing to answer some questions?

If No, terminate
If Yes, continue

Enter the location of this interview

Q1   location?
          1   Location 1   (   )
          2   Location 2   (   )
          3   Location 3   (   )
          4   Location 4   (   )
          5   Location 5   (   )
          6   Location 6   (   )

Q2   Please tell me if you have a pet in your household, and if so, how many of each type of animal? (Circle the appropriate number)

		<1	<2	<3	<4	<5
Q2A	Dog?		(1)	(2)	(3)	(4)	(5)
Q2B	Cat?		(1)	(2)	(3)	(4)	(5)
Q2C	Bird?		(1)	(2)	(3)	(4)	(5)
Q2D	Other Animals?	(1)	(2)	(3)	(4)	(5)

Q3   How long have you had your pet?
          1   Less than 1 year   (   )
          2   1 to 5 years   (   )
          3   Over 5 years   (   )

Q4   How often have you visited your veterinarian in the last year?
          1   Once   (   )
          2   Twice   (   )
          3   Thrice   (   )
          4   More frequently   (   )

Q5   What was the reason for these visits?
          1   Illness   (   )
          2   Vaccination   (   )
          3   Injuries   (   )
          4   Routine treatment   (   )
          5   Health Check   (   )
          6   Operation   (   )
          7   Other   (   )

Q6   On these visits, were any of the following services used or administered on the premises?
          1   X-rays   (   )
          2   Laboratory tests   (   )
          3   ECG test   (   )
          4   Dental work   (   )
          5   Hospital stay   (   )
          6   Other   (   )

Q7a   (without prompting) Which veterinary clinic do you use?

Q7   Which veterinarian do you use?
          1   XYZ Animal Hospital   (   )
          2   Veterinary Practice B   (   )
          3   Veterinary Practice C   (   )
          4   Veterinary Practice D   (   )
          5   Veterinary Practice E   (   )
          6   Veterinary Practice F   (   )
          7   PROMPTING NEEDED   (   )
          8   OTHER – SPECIFY   (   )

Q8   And how did you find this veterinary
       practice?
       1   Personal Recommendation   ( )
       2   Pet store/breeder   ( )
       3   Kennels   ( )
       4   Yellow Pages   ( )
       5   Other local directory   ( )
       6   By chance, off the street   ( )
       7   Other   ( )

Q9   How long have you used this veterinary
       practice?
       1   Less than one year   ( )
       2   1 to 2 years   ( )
       3   2 to 5 years   ( )
       4   Over five years   ( )

Q10   Have you changed your veterinarian
       recently, and if so, why?
       1   No, I have not changed   ( )
       2   Yes, I moved house   ( )
       3   Yes, not satisfied with service   ( )
       4   Yes, not satisfied with price   ( )
       5   Yes, not satisfied with staff   ( )
       6   Yes, not satisfied with the
            veterinarian   ( )
       7   Other   ( )

Q11A Are you aware of other veterinarians in
       the area?
       1   No – go to 12a   ( )   12A
       2   Yes   ( )   11B

Which veterinary clinics in the area are you
aware of?

Q11B Name the other practices
       1   XYZ Animal Hospital   ( )
       2   Name, address veterinarian B ( )
       3   Name, address veterinarian C ( )
       4   Name, address veterinarian D ( )
       5   Name, address veterinarian E ( )
       6   Name, address veterinarian F ( )
       7   OTHER – SPECIFY   ( )

Q12a How do you travel to your veterinary
       clinic?

Q12   How do you travel to your veterinary
       practice?
       1   Car   ( )
       2   Bus/Train/Taxi   ( )
       3   Walk   ( )

13a – On a scale of 1 to 5, where 1 is bad and
5 is very good; how do you rate your present
veterinary clinic on the following attributes?

		Very bad	–	–	–	Very good
Q13A	friendly/helpful receptionist	(1)	(2)	(3)	(4)	(5)
Q13B	friendly/helpful veterinarian	(1)	(2)	(3)	(4)	(5)
Q13C	prompt service	(1)	(2)	(3)	(4)	(5)
Q13D	professional facilities	(1)	(2)	(3)	(4)	(5)
Q13E	clean facilities	(1)	(2)	(3)	(4)	(5)
Q13F	value for money	(1)	(2)	(3)	(4)	(5)
Q13G	availability 24 hours 7 days	(1)	(2)	(3)	(4)	(5)
Q13H	ease of parking?	(1)	(2)	(3)	(4)	(5)

14a – What is important to you in selecting a
veterinarian? Rate the following on a scale of
1 to 5, where 1 is not important and 5 is very
important

		Not important	–	–	–	Very important
Q14A	personality of the veterinarian	(1)	(2)	(3)	(4)	(5)
Q14B	pick-up and delivery service for pets	(1)	(2)	(3)	(4)	(5)
Q14C	friendly/helpful staff	(1)	(2)	(3)	(4)	(5)
Q14D	prompt service	(1)	(2)	(3)	(4)	(5)
Q14E	modern facilities	(1)	(2)	(3)	(4)	(5)

Q14F   special services
on the premises:
x-ray, ECG,
laboratory,
dental, hospital (1) (2) (3) (4) (5)

Q14G   home visits   (1) (2) (3) (4) (5)

Q14H   ease of parking (1) (2) (3) (4) (5)

Do you have a preference for a male or female
veterinarian?

Q15A   Male or female preference?
Q15B   Why?
1   Prefer male   ( )

15B _____
2   Indifferent   ( )

15B _____
3   Prefer female   ( )

15B _____

Do you have a preference for an older or
younger veterinary surgeon?

Q15C   Older or younger preference?
Q15D   Why?
1   Prefer older   ( )

15D _____
2   Indifferent   ( )

16D _____
3   Prefer younger   ( )

15D _____

In your opinion, is there a benefit to having
more than one veterinary surgeon in a clinic?
Would you prefer a multi veterinarian clinic?

Q16A   Would you prefer a clinic with more
than one veterinarian?
1   Yes, prefer multi
veterinarian   ( )
2   Indifferent   ( )
3   No benefit for me   ( )

Q16B   Why?

Q16C   Would you use the nearest clinic to
your house, or would you be prepared
to travel further to another of your
choice?
1   Choose the nearest   ( )
2   Indifferent   ( )
3   Travel further   ( )

Q17   What are the most convenient times of
day to visit your veterinarian?
Specifically,
1   Morning, 8am-1pm   ( )
2   Afternoon, 1pm-5pm   ( )
3   Evening, 5pm-6pm   ( )
4   Evening, 6pm-7pm   ( )
5   Evening, 7pm-8pm   ( )

Q18   Would you be attracted to extra
weekend surgery hours?
1   Saturday afternoon   ( )
2   Saturday evenings   ( )
3   Sunday mornings   ( )

19a – On a scale of 1 to 5 where 1 is a negative
attribute, and 5 is a positive attribute, how
would you rate your veterinarian?

		Very – – – Very		
		negative		**positive**
Q19A	incompetent or competent	(1) (2)	(3)	(4) (5)
Q19B	abrupt or helpful/ obliging	(1) (2)	(3)	(4) (5)
Q19C	rude or polite	(1) (2)	(3)	(4) (5)
Q19D	condescending or reassuring	(1) (2)	(3)	(4) (5)
Q19E	unpleasant or kind to animals	(1) (2)	(3)	(4) (5)
Q19F	short-tempered or patient	(1) (2)	(3)	(4) (5)

Information about the pet owner

Q20   Sex
1   Male   ( )
2   Female   ( )

Q20B	age bracket?		Q20C	income bracket?	
1	Under 16	( )	1	Under 5k	( )
2	17–24	( )	2	6–9k	( )
3	25–34	( )	3	10–13k	( )
4	35–44	( )	4	14–18k	( )
5	45–64	( )	5	19–24k	( )
6	over 65	( )	6	over 25k	( )

Survey Analysis

A computer spreadsheet programme is used to collate and analyse the results and the following notes summarise the range of information which can be prepared and used in the preparation of a detailed marketing plan for the study practice.

Location

The results identify the percentage of respondents at each of the chosen locations and the market share of each of the identified practices in each of the locations.

Distribution of Sample by Pet Ownership

The results identify the spread of pet ownership by species and number throughout the catchment area of the survey and by each of the veterinary practices identified in the survey catchment area.

Length of Pet Ownership

The results identify the period of time owners have owned a pet and compare the results for each of the practices identified in the survey catchment area.

Frequency of Visits

The results identify the number of occasions on which pet owners have visited their veterinarian during the last twelve months and compare the results for each of the practices identified in the survey catchment area.

Reasons for Visits

The results identify the reasons given by pet owners for visiting their veterinarian and compare the results for each of the practices identified in the survey catchment area.

Special Services on the Premises

The results summarise the special services which were perceived by pet owners as being available in each of the veterinary practice premises.

Veterinary Practice Market Share of Sample

The results identify which practice is the market leader on the basis of the survey and the appropriate market share for each of the other practices identified.

Practice Market Share by Location

The results can be used to prepare a matrix to identify the market share position for each of the practices identified at each of the survey locations.

Overview of Market Share Strengths

The results can be used to prepare an overview in market share terms of any or all of the identified practices.

Effectiveness of Practice Promotion

The results can be used to prepare a matrix identifying the extent to which each of the factors identified in question 8 was responsible for promoting any or all of the identified practices.

Loyalty to Veterinary Practice

The results can be used to prepare a matrix identifying the length of time pet owners have been clients of their own veterinarian and thus suggesting the comparative degree of client loyalty which they enjoy.

Reasons for Changing Veterinarian

The results summarise the reasons why pet owners have changed their veterinarian and compare the factors for each of the practices identified and their contribution to the clients decisions to seek advice elsewhere.

Awareness of Other Practices

The results can be used to identify pet owners general awareness of other veterinary practices in the area and for clients of each of the identified practices, their awareness of specific other practices.

Transport

The results can be used to compare the method used by clients to visit their own particular practice with the general means of transport for all the pet owners in the area or for those of any other particular practice in the survey.

Rating Your Present Veterinarian

The results can be used to prepare a matrix to identify the rating for any or all of the practices in the survey in respect of the practice characteristics included in question 13. Usually the results are presented in such a way that the rating for each characteristic for the study practice is compared with the overall sample rating of all the other practices.

Preference for Male or Female Veterinarians

For a variety of reasons some pet owners indicate a preference for a veterinarian of a specific sex. The results can be used to assess any such preference for the clients of all or any of the practices included in the survey.

Age Preference

Similarly some pet owners express a preference for a veterinarian in a specific age group. The results can be used to prepare an analysis of any such preference for the overall sample clients or for the clients of any of the practices specified in the survey.

Preference for Single or Multi Veterinarian Practice

For a variety of reasons some pet owners specify a preference for single handed or multi-veterinarian practices. The results can be used to compare any such preferences which may exist for the overall sample clients or for the clients of any of the practices specified in the survey.

Travel Distance

The results can be used to compare pet owners perceptions of the importance of visiting a veterinary practice which is close to their home and any differences between the views of the overall sample pet owners or for the clients of any of the practices specified in the survey.

Opening Hours

The perceived importance of being able to visit the veterinarian during particular 'office' or 'emergency' hours are revealed by the survey. The results can be used to compare the response from clients of any particular practice with the overall sample response or with the response from clients of any other practice.

Rating Your Present Veterinarian

The results can be used to prepare a matrix which summarises the overall perception of any particular veterinarian in the survey (according to the characteristics incorporated in question 19) with the overall perception of veterinarians in general or with any other specific practice in the area.

Demographic Distribution of Sample

The distribution of pet owners by age and by gender for the whole sample or for the clients of specific practices can be identified and summarised.

Comparison of Current Experience with 'Ideal'

The results in response to questions 13 and 14 can be used to prepare a matrix which compares the current experience of pet owners for any particular criteria with the importance placed on those characteristics (the ideal).

The data is entered into a computer software programme for detailed analysis. The results are used to prepare a marketing profile of the study practice incorporating practice strengths and weaknesses in marketing terms. Comparisons must then clearly be made between the perceived image of the practice in the eyes of existing clients and other pet owners in the locality. The information is then used as the basis for developing an overall marketing strategy and a medium term marketing plan for the practice.

6

The People Who Work in Your Practice

Personnel Management

There can be few areas in practice management which have the potential for so much conflict, misunderstanding and dispute than in personnel management. The handling of relationships with professional veterinarian colleagues, partners or employees can be the most difficult of all.

The two largest costs of delivering veterinary care are those related to staff and drug and professional supplies. The control of these two major expense headings is at the heart of the management role.

Controlling drug and professional supply costs is much the easier of the two. Stock is composed of tangible assets which can be purchased, sold, dispensed or, if damaged or out of date, thrown away. Products can be manipulated, assessed and managed according to their shelf life, cost and efficacy. A drug doesn't talk back. A drug stays where you put it and usually, but not always, does what you expect it to do.

People are not so easy to manage. People talk back. People are late. People have emotions. The value contributed by individuals can't easily be measured. Employers purchase time from their employees but it is not easy to compare an hour of one employee's time with an hour contributed by another. Personnel management requires a great deal of experience, knowledge, communication skills and sensitivity.

All professional practices depend on people to provide the quality of service on which their survival depends. Personnel costs include the costs of recruiting and training staff, fringe benefits, statutory tax, health and other insurance costs, accommodation and a share of overhead and management costs in addition to the specific salary and wage costs of the individuals involved.

Veterinary practice is very labour intensive. Success depends absolutely on the ability of every member of the team including the practice owner(s) to provide the wide range of services that clients require.

Unlike machines, people demand attention, compassion, direction and effort. Practices must educate and train their employees. No new employee arrives at the practice fully prepared to meet the challenges of the position. Training requires a significant investment in time and money to enable employees to reach an acceptable level of competence. The costs of training must be appreciated and budgeted for if the practice is to achieve its potential.

Staff management is a crucial and involved process in even the smallest practice. In larger practices, principals, managers, administrators and lead personnel for each service department (reception, nursing, technician and clerical) may all have varying responsibilities in the development and management of staff. If the level and direction of that responsibility is not clear, confusion can result. The cost will be poor service to clients and ineffective employees. Most veterinary practices are rich in the skills necessary to provide for the medical and surgical management of the patient. The skills required to safeguard the interests of the people who provide those services, and on which the viability of the practice depends, are not always so evident. Perhaps the prime leadership role in veterinary practice should be aimed at preserving the practice's most valuable asset — the stock of hours purchased from employees for service to clients.

Staffing problems are very difficult to disguise and are almost always followed by some sort of communication problem involving clients. A practice with unhappy and unsettled staff is very obvious to clients. An outsider can readily see the difference between a practice with committed, involved staff and one where the sense of harmony and team-work is missing and the staff are more concerned with their personal interests and problems than they are with their job.

Western economies are all being affected by demographic changes which have a marked impact on the profile of the available workforce. The changes in the composition of the population are already substantial and the effects will be far reaching. In the UK for example, one million fewer 16 to 19 year olds in 1994 than 1984, can be expected. The number of people of working age will grow by only half a million between 1989 and 2001, only a quarter of the annual growth rate of the previous decade, and women are expected to account for over 95% of the projected growth of the labour force over the next very few years.

Recruiting and Retaining Staff

One of the most important management tasks for a successful practice principal will be to recognise, recruit and retain talent but it is clear from discussions with many practice principals that personnel management is one of the areas with which they have most difficulty. Many have gained the impression that employers today need employees rather than other way round. The big question seems to be how to recruit and retain staff members who will be as dedicated, work as hard and be as reliable as you are.

Why do people go to work? No two people would offer the same reasons. Understanding what motivates an individual is extremely complex. Probably the closest we can get is to recognise that employers can only create an environment in which their needs match as closely as possible the needs of their employees. They must then use all their communication skills to encourage staff to do what is required, not with the stick or even with the carrot but by triggering a positive wish by the staff to do the job and to do it properly.

What Do They Want?

What are people looking for in their job? Maybe some or all of the following — a living, security, interest, the challenge of a demanding job, appreciation, recognition and an ability to measure and take pride in their own performance.

In our experience, employees want to know what is required, when they are doing well and when there are shortcomings. Money and other benefits are important but given an adequate level of remuneration there is not much evidence that the promise of additional cash on its own is likely to act as a positive motivator to any significant degree.

Good employees deserve to be paid well but the size of the pay cheque is by no means the only factor which employees consider important. The base salary and bonuses are a mere starting point. Working conditions, a sense of belonging, a sense of worth and of being an essential member of the practice family, as well as opportunities for continuing education and for professional advancement will all play a part in an employee's decision to accept or to retain employment in the practice.

For women practitioners, an employer's willingness over and above the requirements of the law, to work around the demands of pregnancy and the subsequent after-care of the baby is a critical selection issue. In some countries, paternity leave is also granted. Open discussion of these issues is essential.

What Don't They Want?

We do know some of the things that staff members don't want. Nursing, technician, clerical, administrative and other support staff want to be known as such. They don't want to be referred to as 'lay staff'. Ask your staff 'what is great about working here?' or 'what are the problems about working here?' The answers will be very revealing. If you are sincere with your questioning and encourage your staff to speak frankly you might hear 'I am treated as though I am of no consequence around here and my contribution is regarded as being of little value'. At a recent series of seminars for reception, clerical and nursing staff held in the UK, many of the delegates told us that they felt underutilised and underappreciated. They positively wanted to be much more involved and increasingly active team members to ensure the success of the enterprise where they spend so much of their working time.

Large organisations spend a significant proportion of their annual budget on personnel management. This includes monitoring staff turnover, exit interviews, recruiting and retention packages, and training and personnel records. Small businesses like veterinary practices should allocate the personnel role to a specific individual such as one of the partners or the practice manager. They must ensure that all the staff records are maintained efficiently, remain confidential and comply with the requirements of the appropriate legislation.

Staff records should include at least the following information:

- name, address and telephone number.
- name and contact telephone number of next of kin.
- advertisement and interview details.
- letters of application and all correspondence.
- previous tax, health insurance and other details.
- contract of employment including a summary of responsibilities, hours, holiday entitlement, sickness and a summary of all absences and holidays during the employment to date.
- a written record of all interviews, particularly if they are disciplinary in nature.

Effective Recruiting

Veterinary practice principals and managers clearly believe that recruiting veterinary graduates is difficult. Grumbling and reminiscing about 'the good old days' is pointless. Each stage in the recruiting process must be taken step by step.

Step 1.

Write down why you want to employ a veterinarian. Is it to allow you to have some time off, to enable you to pursue the growth plans that you have in mind, to open a new practice location or to acquire crucial new professional skills for your clients or to replace an existing employee?

Step 2.

Prepare a detailed job description of the position you will be offering and the personal characteristics you require in your chosen employee. What level of salary package can you afford and what level of professional support are you seeking? Are your expectations realistic? Don't forget that your potential new employee will need to fit in to the existing practice and to identify with your practice philosophy and values. Do not expect to change the nature of people after they have joined your practice. The way they seem on the day of the interview may be (if you are lucky) the way they will seem to your clients on day one of their employment.

The employment must be cost effective. Be sure that the direct and indirect costs of your new employee will be outweighed as quickly as possible by the additional revenue which they generate. Make sure that they realise that they must pay their way in your practice by generating significant additional turnover and by making a positive contribution to the growth of the business. They must be able to communicate well with your existing staff and your clients. Your new recruit must assimilate your practice philosophy and shared values for service readily, to maintain your practice image.

Effective recruiting requires careful preparation. You should;

- identify the required characteristics of the new employee.
- prepare a job description.
- draft, refine and place suitable advertisements.
- prepare a short-list for interview.
- plan how and when you will offer the position to achieve a positive response.
- prepare a letter of appointment incorporating the agreed terms of the contract.
- ensure that you receive a letter confirming acceptance of the position with an agreed start date.
- train, motivate and integrate the new staff member in the practice.

Job Descriptions

Prepare a brief but comprehensive job description for every member of your staff as a pattern, so that you are prepared if and when they have to be replaced. Ask your present staff to write down all the tasks they do and all the jobs which they perceive as their responsibility. What they include or perhaps what is left out may surprise you. Set up a programme for reviewing job descriptions regularly to keep them up to date.

Advertising

You will be competing with many other veterinary practices. They will all try to recruit the best. Create an advertisement to attract interest. Identify your special and unique practice and highlight the career opportunity offered to the successful candidate. Emphasise how the position can satisfy the candidates needs, not yours. Highlight the importance of the successful applicant's career plans, special professional interests, training and continuing professional development requirements. For today's employees, their quality of life, time for leisure and family, career development and opportunities for specialisation may well be more important than a simple financial package.

Interviewing

Allocate enough time to do the job properly. Don't rush it. Try not to interview under pressure and don't talk too much. Overselling the job can create problems later on. Expectations may exceed the reality. You may end up with a dissatisfied short term employee and will soon have to go through the whole process again. Make notes as you go and jot down all the characteristics of the interviewee that you judge to be significant. Remember that 'what you see is what you will get'. Avoid questions which are closed - which only require a yes/no answer. Don't ask questions which may cause legal difficulties later on. Employment law worldwide is becoming more and more complex and you are advised to seek legal advice if in any doubt.

The objectives of the exercise are to

i) acquire by careful questioning as much relevant information about the candidate and pertaining to the position offered as possible.

ii) try to match your needs with the needs of the employee and

iii) once you are satisfied that this candidate may be what you are looking for, to 'sell' the opportunity you are offering so that they will find it hard to say no!

That means asking open-ended questions to encourage the candidate to talk. You are not looking merely for the answers to the questions you pose but an opportunity to assess the candidates attitude to hard work, to their previous employer, to the veterinary profession, to clients, to animals, to other staff members and to the business of veterinary practice. Here are a few examples of good questions — but don't use them all every time!:

Some Questions

- Tell me about your last job, your pets and experience with animals.
- What did you like best in your last job?
- How could you have improved your performance in your last job?
- How did you get on with your boss, your colleagues and your subordinates in your last job?
- How would they score your performance?
- Tell me about one of the things that gave you most pride in your last job?
- Did you receive the recognition you deserved in your previous job?
- What didn't you like in your last job, what went wrong, why did you leave?
- Tell me about the best boss you've ever had?
- Tell me about the worst boss you've ever had.
- What do you think is your greatest strength?
- Do you like a job with a lot of responsibility and/or one with a lot of freedom?
- Have you ever made a poor judgement? — tell me what you would do now, in similar circumstances.
- How do you feel about euthanasia for animals?
- How would you handle the following situation? — be specific.
- Tell me what your referee will tell me about you when I phone him.

Try not to shut off the candidate when he replies — keep his comments coming by responding with a further comment or question — that's interesting, tell me about it, why?, how? and so on.

Ask your existing staff members to help in the selection process. Take the opportunity of walking together through the practice and introducing the candidate to your staff. Afterwards have a word with them to assess their instant judgment. Don't forget that your clients will make such judgments and you should be aware of the potential impact of the candidate on them and on your existing staff team.

The final stage of the interview is perhaps the most crucial. You will probably have divided the candidates into a number of categories including the:

- 'no — not under any circumstances' group
- 'the possibles — worth thinking about' group and
- 'the probables — first impressions very favourable' group.

Wind up the interview in a business like way so that both parties understand how the situation is left and who is to make the next move. Indicate to the 'no hopers' that you are planning to see a number of other candidates and that you will write to them within a specified number of days. Keep your promise. Write, thanking them for their interest but indicate that the position is now filled. As far as the 'possibles' and the 'probables' are concerned, gently probe to assess and encourage their interest in the job. Ask them to consider the possibility of joining the practice and to let you know by telephone whether they would wish to be considered within two days. In this way you will hopefully be left with a short list of candidates who positively want the job.

Make your decision and offer the job verbally to your first choice. If it is accepted confirm your offer in writing that day. Ask for a formal letter of acceptance by return. As soon as the agreement is struck in writing by both parties, write a letter of thanks and regrets to the other candidates.

The Perfect Employee

Recruiting quality members of staff who can quickly absorb the practice philosophy and values for service requires particular skills. Retaining them once they have joined the practice is not automatic. The ongoing personnel management task is to maintain and build upon their initial enthusiasm and maintain their dedication to the practice. Some employees will be happy to be hardworking members of the team from the start. A few will have a degree of entrepreneurial spirit and will need to be treated as special if their creative drive is not to be stifled. The challenge is to take that entrepreneurial spirit and foster its development towards a common good to generate profit for the practice.

The trick then is not to seek employees who are simply compliant but to recognise those who might initially be perceived as rebels but who could be transformed, with good leadership, into departmental or practice leaders of the future. These are the individuals who are excited by a challenge. If their enthusiasm for innovative ideas is matched by their clinical and communication skills, these are the people to nurture. Delegate responsibility to them to plan and develop a new marketing initiative or service development. Be tough and demanding but don't be negative or you might extinguish the creative spark which your practice needs.

Any business requires a staff composed of a mix of individuals with differing levels of skill, experience and knowledge to create a balanced whole. So it is with personalities. Can you imagine how disastrous it might be if all the employees were rebels, innovative and entrepreneurial? Some practice managers use personality profile tests as part of the interviewing process. A number of them are available commercially. They can be conducted and interpreted by a suitably qualified employee of the licensed vendor. Understanding an individual's personality type and their response to dominance, influence, steadfastness, and discipline standards gives you a good indication of how they would function within your practice.

Whether or not additional personality testing tools are used, the intuition and common sense of the individual conducting the interview is crucial. The best interviewers spend much more time listening than talking. Listening is an active task. It requires a considerable degree of concentration to hear, understand and interpret what is said by the candidate. If the interviewee sounds negative, judgmental or reserved, consider why they are taking a less than positive attitude. Perhaps the pressure of the interview is distorting their true personality. Perhaps what you see and hear is what you will get. By all means look hard to find the good points but dont make the mistake of believing that your practice is a reclamation service for inappropriate employees as well as sick animals. You may be good at the second. You probably will not be so effective at the first.

Once you have agreed to employ this special entrepreneurial individual you must consider a strategy to make the best use of them. An employed entrepreneur may be described as an 'intrapreneur'.

Intrapreneurs have wonderful ideas but hate to document them. They can be excellent clinicians, are often worshipped by clients but hate sticking to the business discipline required by the practice manager. Money may motivate these individuals but their biggest motivation is generated by the challenges which face them. They become bored when the challenge is met and the trick for the employer is to encourage the intrapreneur to identify new challenges and attain new targets while continuing the task for which they have been employed.

The symbiotic relationship between a veterinary practice and the employees which operate it must be readily understood by every single member of the staff. Owners and employees will recognise that both parties must benefit from the relationship which can only prosper if the practice is profitable. Employees sometimes find it difficult to understand the need for profit. The practice principal, manager or director should make it their business to allocate time to talk to their staff about the issue. The message is a very simple one. This practice will not be able to continue to provide a quality level of professional veterinary services unless it makes money. The more money it makes, the more it is able to distribute amongst the staff. The more it is able to invest in continuing education, equipment, facilities and services, the happier will be the clients and the more it will grow.

Keeping Your Staff

Recruiting replacement staff is an expensive business. A crucial part of your personnel plan will relate to your policies for retaining the staff you already have. How much you are prepared to pay for their on-going services will be an important but probably not their over-riding consideration. Talk to your staff, find out what matters are of concern to them and see if you can match their needs with those of your practice.

They will almost certainly want a realistic financial package as well as a position and a role in your practice which can provide them with job satisfaction.

Remuneration

The level of remuneration offered to an employee is likely to be a major matter for discussion. The value of the total compensation package is likely to include a basic salary, bonuses, payroll taxes, medical benefits, housing or other accommodation costs, pension, use of cars, deferred options for shares (in those countries where incorporation of veterinary practice is possible) and possibly an additional performance related component. The question of tax liability for employer or employee must also be clarified and the advice of the practice accountant should be sought in this respect. In some countries the law will require the value of fringe benefits to be liable to tax. In others, such benefits must be non-discriminatory and may not be negotiated with one party to the exclusion of another. Practice principals should seek legal advice if they are in any doubt.

A base salary with a possibility of a future bonus is probably the most appropriate method of compensation for a newly qualified graduate. Some employers are keen to base the salary on a percentage of gross income collected. Before considering such an option, potential employees should have sufficient experience to charge properly for services and to judge the financial health of the practice, the type of clientele, the competence of the other staff, the fee levels, the equipment and level of medicine being practised and the current case volume. All of these factors will have an impact on the likely level of revenue which the veterinarian will be able to generate. Such a system may be an excellent performance based procedure for determining an appropriate salary but not, we think, for a new graduate.

For a new graduate the best approach is to negotiate a guaranteed salary. If the employee's performance becomes exemplary and outstanding, the possibility of a bonus payment should be available and should be based on the practice owner's opinion of the employee's total contribution to the practice. Bonuses should be offered sparingly. If every employee receives a bonus every month the exercise becomes meaningless and employees simply regard the bonus as part of their base salary. For the bonus to be meaningful it must be based upon exceptional and occasional standards of service beyond that normally anticipated and required.

Exceptional standards of performance may be based upon;

- gross income collected, perhaps excluding the sale of low profit margin merchandised items.
- the number of man hours spent in the practice during the year.
- the number of particular transactions generated by the employee.
- the employee's commitment to help support staff or to assist in their training.
- the employee's involvement in administrative tasks such as assisting in the planning and institution of a computer system or a new stock control system.
- the employees willingness to volunteer personal time to monitor the health of cases assigned to him and others in the practice.

All of these are examples of performance above and beyond the call of duty and should be recognised and rewarded accordingly.

Salary levels for veterinarians vary widely within individual countries and throughout the world. The demographic makeup of the area, the cost of living, hours demanded for the professional's time, the type of practice (equine, small animal, mixed practice, cattle and so on), fee structure and many other factors will have a bearing on the amount that an employer can offer an employee veterinarian. Salary levels will also depend on the supply and demand of veterinarians in the marketplace. In most countries the appropriate professional veterinary association accumulates and monitors salary levels for veterinary professionals as a guide to employers and employees alike.

Times change. Practitioners who graduated in the sixties and seventies accepted that their time off would be limited. They knew that it was expected that their career came first, well ahead of family and leisure. In recent years veterinarians have recognised the importance of quality of life and enough free time to pursue hobbies, spend more time with family and develop ancillary interests. They are now much more likely to question the total hours that they should be available for their practice commitments. Increasingly, it will be necessary to identify these responsibilities in the contract of employment. What was once thought to be an unspoken expectation now becomes a contractual requirement.

The Financial Package

A fair and equitable salary is a subjective perception. Make sure that the total financial package provides a good basic salary with some provision for employee performance to enhance it.

Veterinarians operate a number of systems for determining salary levels. Some employees receive a fixed salary on a time commitment basis i.e. for so many hours per week and weeks per year. The terms need to be clear, identifying holiday entitlement, paid periods for continuing education and with an indication of how frequently and when the figure will be reviewed.

The other approach used by some practices, particularly for professional veterinary staff, is based on performance, either linked to gross revenue generated by the individual or linked in some way to profit. The rules have to be set and agreed to at the outset. How do you deal, for example, with bad debtors and over the counter sales? What happens if veterinarian A generates a great deal of surgical work which is then dealt with by veterinarian B? One advantage of the profit sharing approach is that it does overcome the problem of paying on the basis of a high turnover but with many slow or bad payers. On the other hand it implies that you must identify what you mean by profit and how it is determined. There is no reason at all why an employee who accepts a higher salary should not be reminded that they also have to accept a responsibility to generate the additional turnover required to pay for it.

In the United States a fair return for a veterinarian employee is 20% to 22% of the fees earned and collected (excluding OTC sales and food products). Fringe benefits may add up to an additional 30% of the basic salary (continuing education, professional subscriptions, private motoring and accommodation).

Productivity

The performance related part of the package will depend on the individual's productivity. You will need to consider a number of ways of measuring performance for professional and non-professional staff. What are the bench marks? How much would you expect your professional staff to generate in fee and medication sales £80,000, £100,000, £120,000, £150,000 or are we pitching these figures too high or too low? What do you think?

How else could you measure productivity, case volume, average transaction value, organisational ability, team spirit, ability to generate business, to retain clients, to achieve improved responses to clinical reminders or to reduce complaints? The possibilities are endless and you will need to consider what is appropriate for your practice and for your staff.

'FREEBIES' How do you overcome the problem of veterinary staff who give away too many 'free' consultations because they are not as aware as you are, of what it costs the practice. One suggestion might be to give new professional staff a cash sum, say £100 per month for the first few months, which they could use as they wished. But, they would have to pay the practice for the consultations they wanted to give away free. Anything left at the end of the month is theirs to keep.

Performance Related Pay

One of the perceived advantages from the employer's point of view in determining a salary level based on a percentage of the gross revenue generated by the practice or individual employee, is that it will eliminate the stress of salary negotiations in future years. Employers may think that the percentage will be an automatic inducement for employees to excel. The employees may, however, view the situation differently and will probably wish to see salary increases over and above that related to improved productivity. Within a limited range this is probably reasonable. Employees become less of a hassle to a practice as their productivity increases and their experience may be expected to result in fewer clinical or communication difficulties. In addition, the employee veterinarian may be invaluable in advising and training less experienced veterinarians and other employees in the practice. They may also have made some other real contribution to the profitability of the practice but which may not necessarily result in a significant increase in the individuals gross revenue.

A number of complications and possible abuses can occur however, and we recommend that new employees should not be paid on the basis of individual gross turnover until they have had an opportunity of demonstrating their value to the practice by working on a fixed salary basis for a probationary period of say, six months.

There are other possibilities. Some practices have found that automatic year-end bonuses are an effective way to motivate employee veterinarians. On the other hand, bonuses that are anticipated and expected by the employee are too often perceived simply as a way of deferring a sum which should be regarded as part of the base salary. Under these circumstances, the bonus system may be counter productive and of little or no value as a motivational tool.

Discretionary bonuses, on the other hand, provide employers with a pooling formula designed to protect the profit margin and to establish an incentive system for employees. A pre-determined pool of money, based as a percentage of fees, is set aside and used to pay bonuses at the year end. The employer is not committed to distributing all of the money within the pool and this allows considerable flexibility to allocate resources to individual employees which are judged to have made a significant contribution, which may or may not include simple financial measures, to the success of the practice.

This system too, is not without possible problems. It depends on the subjective judgement of the employer or manager. His judgement may be clouded by personal prejudices and he may have an unfair bias for or against a particular employee. The problem here is the perception of the value of that judgement by the other employees. It is not difficult to imagine a situation in which the bonus scheme is abandoned because its basis falls into disrepute.

The whole question of bonus distribution, discretionary or otherwise, depends on the individual practice philosophy. Not every circumstance demands the same solution. Individual judgement is critical in determining the most appropriate system for any particular practice to reward key people. The success of any bonus system depends on a fair and equitable distribution of any resources which are available. Some employees have provided far greater service and as such should be rewarded with a larger share of the pool. Some employees should not even be considered for a bonus. Mediocre performance by one or more individuals which is rewarded with a bonus payment is likely to have a devastating impact on the morale of the other hard-working, productive employees in the practice.

A performance based system which combines a specified salary that anticipates likely levels of production together with an opportunity for employee veterinarians to earn a discretionary bonus, contingent not only on their individual productivity but also on the overall practice performance is preferred for appropriate employees. A financial package based solely on a percentage of gross revenue is not recommended because a number of factors other than the skill or dedication of the veterinarian may contribute to that growth. Refurbishing or reequiping the premises, increasing the numbers of support staff and introducing and installing veterinary computer packages, may all have a dramatic impact on the fee income of the entire practice and the capacity of each individual veterinarian to produce a greater level of gross. In these circumstances the management decisions taken by the practice owner or manager will have a greater impact on turnover than the efforts of the veterinarian employees. Bonus payments paid under these circumstances may at first sight still result in increased profitability but could endanger profit margins in the longer term.

Bonuses should be based upon extra effort and should not be regarded as a means of supplementing an existing salary level. If the employee contributes average or mediocre effort, the chosen system must ensure that no bonus is paid. It must be the responsibility of the practice manager or practice owner to maintain an unbiased, open-minded and up to date knowledge of the contribution made by each of the employees. The ideal employee veterinarian is the one whose experience, knowledge, and medical acumen is reflected in both their ability to generate income and their willingness to contribute to the efficient operation of the practice.

Employers should think long and hard before offering compensation deals to veterinarian employees which are based on bonuses in respect of income generated by the individual over and above a base. Today's revenue levels may be regarded as adequate to service all the practice costs. A marginal salary increase resulting from the additional revenue generated by an enthusiastic employee may be perceived as a fair price to pay. The situation may change considerably, however, within a very few months and for a variety of reasons the new revenue level may then be regarded as a norm. It may then be much easier to achieve because of new fee scales, a newly established merchandising policy or the provision of a new piece of equipment which may have increased the potential fee income to a level which would have been exceptional only a short time earlier. A commitment to continuing bonus payments to an employee under these circumstances may not be cost effective.

We argue elsewhere in this book that the control of cash has become an overriding priority for managers as veterinary practice continues to grapple with recession. Any performance based bonus system should, therefore, be based on fees collected and not fees earned. You should make it quite clear that the employee becomes responsible not only for the delivery of the service but also the collection of the fees involved.

A base salary plus an agreed performance based incentive arrangement seems to be more appropriate and popular as veterinarian employees gain in medical and surgical expertise and in their communication skills with clients. The terms of the agreement for such an arrangement must be documented and included in or attached to the employee's contract of employment. The methodology of calculating bonus payments must be clearly identified with example calculations to ensure that no misunderstandings arise between employer and employee on the issue. As practice situations change, additional arrangements or amendments to the agreement can be attached on an annual basis.

Experienced clinicians are sometimes employed on the basis of no fixed base salary with all remuneration being based on the level of fees generated and collected. Each practice has a different profit margin so the appropriate relationship between the fees collected and the salary earned will vary similarly. If the employee veterinarian can contribute in improving the practice's profit margin, then there may be a greater justification for offering a more generous percentage compensation arrangement. The employee has an opportunity to improve his income, not only by working harder but also by working more efficiently and effectively and by conserving operating costs.

Overtime Compensation

In many countries, time worked in excess of a specified number of hours (e.g., 40 hours) may entitle some groups of employees to receive a premium payment for the additional work. In the UK and the US, overtime payment is not generally paid to employee veterinarians because of the tradition of their professional status. Some practices provide compensatory time off for their professional staff members who have contributed a great deal of overtime in excess of the hours specified in the contract of employment. Specific time off clauses may be included within the employment contract as a separate inducement to employees to excel. It is much more common for the employer to offer, at his discretion, time off as and when it is possible. In most

instances, however, employees seem to prefer bonus payments rather than compensatory time off.

It is sensible to include some reference to working hours and pro rata arrangements in the contract of employment for all staff members including veterinarians. Most small animal practitioners in the United States work a minimum of 45 to 50 hours per week in order to practice their profession and maintain a level of service for the practice's patients. The time span is even more demanding in large animal practices at anywhere from 45 to 55 hours per week and veterinarians in the UK, for example, would not regard these figures as exceptional.

The appropriate compensation arrangements for any particular practice or employee, clearly depends on the particular circumstances which exist. Both parties need to examine those circumstances with care. In any employer/employee relationship, the role of the employee is to convince the employer that he is worthy of a respectable salary. The role of the employer is to pay a salary which is clearly equitable and fair, and to provide a working environment in which the employee can justify that salary level.

Employment Agreements

Employers and employees are likely to have different and potentially opposing interests in the practice. Both parties will need to negotiate terms which are acceptable to both and, as in all negotiations, the happiest outcome occurs when both parties perceive themselves as 'winners'. Employer and employee should seek to appreciate and understand each others objectives and work to meet the common good. Usually, this understanding is documented in the form of an agreement or contract between the two individuals.

The law which relates to employment varies considerably from country to country. Employers must ensure that the employment contract, written or verbal, complies with the specific statutory requirements which may apply. The agreement should certainly;

- identify the parties.
- include the job title.

- specify the date when employment began (if the employment is for a fixed term, the expiry date must also be included).
- the rate of pay or the method by which pay is calculated, and the pay period (hourly, weekly or monthly).
- normal working and specific rules which may apply.
- entitlement to holidays including public holidays and rates of holiday pay.
- rules on sickness or injury absence and sick pay
- details of pension scheme if appropriate.
- the length of notice the employee is entitled to receive and must give.
- any disciplinary rules in operation.
- a person to whom the employee can take any grievance.

Reference may be given to circumstances which will be regarded as gross misbehaviour justifying termination of the employment without notice. The contract should also include reference to other disciplinary procedures and to steps which the employee may take in case of grievance. Legal advice should always be sought by either party and employers must comply with the employment legislation current in the country in which they operate.

Responsibilities and Duties

The required responsibilities and duties of the employee must be clearly identified. In the past it has been sufficient to indicate that 'the duties will be those normally accepted by a veterinarian in clinical practice'. Today, however, detailed requirements should be specified. If, for example, the veterinarian's duties require that they be available for work at 8:00 in the morning and leave at 7:00 p.m., except on those occasions when they are on duty overnight, that obligation should be clearly identified in the agreement. It may or may not assist either party in case of a subsequent dispute but at the very least its inclusion ensures that the matter has been discussed, debated and agreed by both parties at the outset.

Confidentiality

Total confidentiality in the handling of client and patient information is of critical importance if the public is to rely on the level of discretion by the practice employees. Not only may the employee veterinarian be subject to possible litigation for an indiscreet comment about a particular client but the employer, too, may be responsible for the employee's behaviour under the master/servant doctrine. Accordingly, most employment agreements provide specifically that the privacy of information is sacrosanct thus offering some arguable degree of defence to the employer if action is brought by an aggrieved client.

Other Considerations

The contract of employment may include clauses which refer to compensation issues in addition to those required by the law, in the event of disability, death, or premature termination. The employer may specify how employees are expected to dress and to conduct themselves in a professional manner, as well as conforming to certain codes of ethics which are generally accepted within the veterinary profession. The employer may also wish to insist that the employee maintain certain levels of continuing education, engage in community activities for the benefit of the practice, not accept employment with other employers either veterinary or otherwise or restrict certain personal habits on the premises, such as smoking, that affect the well being of others.

The agreement may also refer to the rights of the employee, including such matters as minimum standards for working conditions, use of secretarial staff, use of telephones, practice vehicles and so on.

Negotiating and Re-negotiating the Contract

Employers and employees should allocate plenty of time to negotiate or renegotiate the terms of the contract. The equivalent of placing a gun to someone's head and saying 'sign' is not likely to be effective. Both parties would be wise to anticipate that the process of negotiation and agreement will take some time. The essence of successful negotiation, it is said, is that both parties are perceived as winners. Neither party will gain in the long run if one 'wins' while the other 'loses'.

It is essential that employees are formally appraised by the employer on a regular basis and that ample time is given to discuss and agree their strengths and weaknesses in the practice. An open and honest exchange of views will strengthen the relationship and both parties will benefit.

Occasionally, memories of what was said or agreed some time after the event do not coincide and there is a powerful argument for documenting the topics covered and the points agreed, perhaps on a proforma, signed by both parties and with a copy for each.

A good employer will help his employees to be good employees; and *vice versa*! The task is time consuming. Personnel management in a practice with a number of employees is not a task which can be undertaken successfully without the provision of adequate time and care. Effective two way communication between employer and employee is as important to the success of veterinary practice as that between the practice and its clients.

Employers must assess the worth of the employee by more than just their ability to serve clients and their patients competently. The future of the business depends on the employee's ability to add a new dimension to the business. The provision of a barely adequate level of service by an employee of a practice which has built a reputation for excellence can rapidly destroy an image which may have taken years to build. You are judged by the company you keep. Choose your associates wisely.

Additional terms of employment which may be implied but not necessarily included in the employment agreement are sometimes found in ancillary documents such as a practice manual for employees. Employees may sometimes accept additional restrictions or responsibilities if they are compensated by additional remuneration, bonuses or other fringe benefits. The subsequent interpretation of the terms of the agreement and the degree to which it may be enforced by either party may be a matter for debate. At the very

least, the discipline implied in seeking agreement ensures that both parties carefully consider all the issues before they sign a contract.

Both parties should enter the agreement enthusiastically and freely and with the intention of respecting the spirit as well as the details of the contract between them. The essence of being a professional depends on accepting some sort of code of professional conduct. It is clearly not practical to include every single aspect of a professional appointment in a formal contract of employment. The document must be fair to both individuals. If it is not, the relationship between professionals will just not work. An employment agreement is of value to both parties because it identifies specific points of contractual obligation but is not confined to them.

Keep the Contract Current

Situations change. The employment agreement between employer and employee must recognise the need for review on a regular basis and for updating as necessary. Sometimes circumstances outside the control of the parties, e.g., changes in the law, may affect the terms of the agreement and we believe that the contract should be dusted down and re-examined on an annual basis at least. Legal advice should be sought by both parties. We acknowledge that such advice can on occasions be so detailed and probing that it kills an arrangement provisionaly agreed by both parties. There is little doubt that the risk of entering a complex contract of employment without professional advice would be even greater.

The employment agreement should include a clause which identifies title to the practice assets. Most contracts, for example, confirm that the efforts of the employee are being compensated by the salary paid and that they are not entitled to gain any equity rights in the practice goodwill or in the client or patient records.

In some countries, it is common practice for potential partners to be offered a discount in respect of their purchase of a share in the practice valuation because of the contribution they have made to generate additional revenue and enhance profitability. This will be a matter for negotiation however, at the time partnership prospects are discussed. It would not normally be wise to include any reference to such proposals in the contract of employment even though it may be the wish of both parties at that time to negotiate a partnership at some future date.

Wherever possible, the terms of the agreement between an employee veterinarian and an employer should be agreed and concluded prior to the commencement of employment. If this is not possible by force of circumstances it is recommended that, at the very least, there should be an exchange of letters between the parties incorporating the major points which they intend to be included in the contract.

Binding Out Clauses

One of the most critical sections in an employment agreement is to ensure that the ownership of client files, patient records and practice goodwill remains firmly in the hands of the employer. It is necessary, therefore, to include a clause which restricts an employee, during the period of employment or subsequently, from competing with the employer within a specified geographical area for a specified period of time.

The law, in this respect, varies from country to country. It is generally believed that the courts will only enforce such provisions if they are perceived to be reasonable. Clearly then, a binding out clause will need to be determined in such a way that it is no more restrictive than is reasonably necessary to protect the interests of the employer while not unreasonably restraining the freedom of the employee to practice his profession. Solutions involving drawing concentric circles on the map and studies which identify areas of 'client draw' have been developed in some countries. In most parts of the world the appropriate professional body will be prepared to offer advice in this respect. We recommend that additional legal advice is a wise investment for both parties.

Distance is only one issue. Time is the second. It is clearly reasonable to restrict a former employee from seeking clients in a catchment area close to that served by his former employer. On the other hand, it is not reasonable to exert such a restriction for the rest of his professional career.

It is, therefore, necessary to incorporate a time limit on any such restriction. Most binding out agreements span anywhere from two to five years. Two to three years seems to be the most common. Binding out agreements for buy-sell agreements are usually very much longer because of the equity relationship between the former owner and the practice.

Non-competition agreements can be exceedingly complex to establish and even more problematical to enforce. Some veterinarians have considered alternative and apparently easier approaches. Instead of agreeing to an appropriate distance and time, the employer merely requires the employee to sign an agreement that he, upon departure from the practice, will not solicit nor serve the specific clients of the employer as from the date of the termination.

Simplicity, however, breeds inaccuracy. The identification and 'safeguarding' of specific clients at a specific point in time will not ensure that the practice's goodwill will be preserved. Most small animal veterinary practices have a response rate for their vaccination reminder systems of somewhere between 50%-70%. This means that anywhere from 30% to 50% of a practice's client base is replenished or renewed on an annual basis. The benefit then of merely preventing a former employee from taking those clients who are currently with the practice is likely to be limited.

Not every employee exhibits the loyalty of a Bob Cratchitt nor every employer the cruelty of an Ebeneezer Scrooge, yet, elements of these personality types exist in many practices. Long-term employees who have given consistent, faithful service to an employer over many years do not have an equity interest in the business. At the same time they have made a major commitment in time and effort in serving their employer and the practice clients. It may seem fair and just they should have an opportunity of deriving some tangible benefit from that commitment.

A number of options have been developed, particularly in the United States, to offer employees such benefits. An employer may, for example, offer a contract to an employee by which, if the employee agrees to work in the practice for a minimum of say, five more years he will receive a specified capital sum equivalent to say six months salary. If the employee's contract is terminated prematurely by the employer, a capital sum will be payable which reflects an appropriate proportion of the original. An alternative arrangement would be for an employee who remains with the employing practice for a specified period to be granted subsequently, a right to practice in competition with the previous employer in return for the payment of a capital sum. Such payment could be made over a period of time and would help to achieve an amicable arrangement which could be of benefit to both parties.

Option to Purchase Equity Interest

The 'American Dream' of eventually acquiring an equity interest in a business is not restricted to Americans. Many veterinarian employees do purchase an equity share in a partnership in due course. In those countries where corporate status for a veterinary practice is permissable, employees are able to make a financial investment in the practice by purchasing or being offered stock in the business in which they work without the obligations of a partner. In such circumstance, an option to purchase an equity interest in a successful practice may be regarded as a significant and valuable form of compensation.

Support Staff

Most veterinary practices employ a number of other staff apart from veterinarians. They are likely to include some or all of the following; technicians, nurses, managers, receptionists, clerical staff, kennel and cleaning staff and so on. Support staff costs in many practices range between 14% to 16% of gross although practices that provide a significant level of additional services such as diagnostic work may incur support staff salaries up to 18% or 20% of turnover.

The allocation of this sum to different support staff groups varies enormously from practice to practice. For example, a particular practice may allocate 6.5% of total gross income to receptionists, 8% of gross income for nurse/technicians, 3% of gross income for the office manager and clerical staff and 2.5% of gross income for kennel and other miscellaneous assistance. In another practice the ranges of percentages will differ. In an individual practice, however, there are advantages in maintaining some consistency in the allocation of resources to the different support staff categories. The manager's role then is to determine how best to utilise the particular pool of money allocated to, say, nursing staff determined by a particular percentage of practice revenue. This will enable him to make a judgement between employing, say, two well paid experienced nurses, three nurses at a lower salary or five part-time individuals. The question for the individual practice is which option will enable the business to operate at its optimum level to achieve the objectives set. The manager will need to remember that nothing stays static for long. Three less experienced nurses this year are likely to have developed into three highly experienced and more expensive employees in two or three years time and a medium term strategy must be determined to ensure that costs are contained within the budgeted category limit throughout the period.

If the support staff recognise that continued practice success depends on maintaining salary levels within category heads as a percentage of revenue generated, there are a number of advantages. They will understand for example, that if they complain that there is too much work for the present staffing, the cost of additional employees will decrease the possibility of salary increases for the more experienced persons.

If management avoids the responsibility of determining individual salary levels according to their perceived value to the practice within categories of staff members, problems can arise. Hardworking and motivated employees will have their incentive to excel destroyed if mediocrity is rewarded at the same level as excellence. Discretion must be given to the manager to manage. He must assess the merits of each individual employee intelligently and negotiate an appropriate salary level within the agreed range. We believe that salary levels should not be determined simply by some computer spreadsheet programme. Creativity and ingenuity, dedication and hard work must be rewarded. If not, the practice will find that dedicated, motivated and resourceful employees will flee to neighbouring colleagues, while the mediocre employees are retained in an increasingly decaying practice.

Salary Levels

A mutual agreement about payment for services rendered is at the heart of the relationship between employer and employee. The difficulties involved in reaching such agreement become more complex every year. For practices of any size it is just not sensible now for the practice principal to make snap decisions about individual remuneration or total compensation packages and expect on the one hand that the staff will be totally satisfied and on the other, that performance will not be affected. It is usually necessary for an individual practice member, possibly a partner or the practice manager, to be responsible for all personnel matters including the question of determining and agreeing salary and total compensation levels.

The adequacy and quality of the staff will largely determine the quality of the service your practice is able to deliver. Staffing cuts to the heart of practice. A veterinary practice does not exist in isolation. It must compete as an employer with large industrial and commercial organisations as well as with other small businesses in the locality. The best practices need top talent. A practice which wishes to offer the best cannot afford to employ anybody but the best. The best employees have a good self image, they seek and will earn a good salary and your personnel and financial plans must incorporate a commitment to pay for the best.

Veterinarians have always been prepared to travel to find the professional experience, the lifestyle and the level of remuneration they seek. Nowadays too, highly trained nursing, technician and other support staff members are also prepared to travel to find the ideal job. Hospital directors and practice managers therefore must remain abreast of terms and conditions of employment throughout the profession if they are to remain competitive.

One of the important roles of national or local professional veterinary associations is to survey and monitor current salary levels and total remuneration packages for a number of professional and support staff employees in veterinary practice. One or two national and international veterinary business publications also monitor and publish such information which is of considerable value in guiding veterinarians and their staff in negotiating appropriate salary levels.

The ancillary costs of employing the best personnel can be considerable and must be taken into account in planning. They include not only statutory elements such as the employer's contribution to employee health insurance and other taxes but also the costs of recruiting and retaining the individual staff members, an appropriate share of the overhead costs and the specific costs of training and continuing professional development.

Keeping Salaries Competitive

The ability of your practice to recruit and pay for the best of employees is related directly to your profitability. The veterinary profession has not been alone in falling victim to the economic pressures in the late 1980's and early 1990's. A practice owner's ability to pay appropriate salary levels is limited by the profit margin inherent within the profession. The pool of resources available for distribution to the staff is not endless but should stay constant as a percentage of gross income. If employee costs as a percentage of gross increase, the profit margin declines and the income of the equity owners of the practice will fall.

In recent years a number of practices, largely because of inadequate management accounting monitoring of costs, have attempted to reverse the erosion of profit margins caused by rising salary levels by severely trimming the other cost headings. This can result in difficulties in other areas of activity and have an impact on the quality of the services offered to clients. The only sensible approach in such matters is to budget carefully, to ensure that the overall cost of employees is maintained within a predetermined percentage of gross, to monitor actual expenditure at frequent intervals and to take corrective action when it is necessary.

If veterinarian employers want to pay their

employees more, they must ensure that sufficient additional gross revenue is generated to pay them. The logic is inescapable. Practice growth usually does not just happen fortuitously. There are exceptions, such as an epidemic of a preventable disease or the collapse of a competing practice, but usually growth must be planned. Marketing strategies, fee schedules and other policies must be designed and implemented for growth.

The first two lessons that any new employee should learn in your practice are;

- Their role is to win and keep new clients for your practice and
- Their salary is directly related to the level of fees which are paid to the practice by those clients.

If these lessons are learned well by your staff they will welcome proposals to increase fees and generate additional revenue. An employee who resists fee increases or who is not prepared to give them whole hearted endorsement in discussing such issues with clients is not likely to receive a salary increase and, in the longer term, will probably not be working for you at all.

Paying employees more must, most definitely, not be done at the expense of the employer. If employees perceive that they can be paid more without producing more, the practice may enter a downward spiral. Performance declines, costs increase, profit margins are eroded, the employer becomes disillusioned and stale and the practice is in decline — soon to be replaced by a new or existing competitor in the market. In comparison with other comparably skilled professions, veterinary medicine generates a relatively low level of return on investment.

Motivation

Good employees are created, not born. A fair salary for an honest day's work recognises an individual's talents to fulfil the responsibilities of the job and to work well with their colleague employees.

Employers employ a variety of tactics in search of a magical formula to motivate employees to perform at the peak of their ability. Incentive

arrangements for support staff have recently been gaining popularity in the veterinary profession. If all workers were autonomous, self-employed contractors, payment determined on the basis of performance would probably make most sense. Employment in the twentieth century however, is largely based upon team effort and not individual achievement. Most successful organisations of any size look to groups of achievement oriented individuals to achieve their objectives and not the one or two lone stars who try to perform beyond the norm at the expense of their fellow workers. This approach too is likely to be the most successful in the business of veterinary practice. Because veterinary practices employ anything from one to fifty or more employees (most employing fewer than ten), the efforts of every individual have a direct bearing upon the results and success of every other person within the group.

Incentive arrangements attempt to gloss over the holistic relationship amongst employees by segregating job functions into pigeon hole activities. Rarely are incentive arrangements perceived as equitable. Unlike the single product businesses of years ago, the successful practice of veterinary medicine usually depends on the efforts of several individuals. Practice owners and managers cannot afford the luxury of letting employees lapse into demarcation disputes.

Practice owners have experimented with a wide range of incentive schemes for support staff members. For some technicians or nursing staff, practices have instituted incentive arrangements based on specific job functions (e.g. the number of dental procedures completed) while some receptionists receive an incentive based upon the number of new clients they have influenced to make an appointment. These staff may be rewarded as piece meal workers at anywhere from $2.50 to $10.00 for each new client (defined as one who has not been to the practice for a number of years).

Sometimes employees learn to manipulate the system to increase their take home pay and may resort to extraordinary salesmanship efforts to meet the quota and receive the bonus. Individual receptionists or nurses may receive commission payments for 'over the counter' or other nonprescription sales. Unless managed with considerable care, this can result in unacceptable pressures on clients, and staff to compromise on their ideals.

Perhaps the best approach to a performance related pay package, particularly for support staff, combines a basic salary sum (perhaps 75% of the total) with an individual performance related element (say 25%) and an additional bonus based on practice results for 'the target for the month' (an opportunity of earning an extra say 5%). The bonus element must be perceived as something extra earned by the individual or by the team but not to be relied on as merely a part of the base. The bonus sum could depend on a number of variables and it will be your management role to decide what is most appropriate for your practice. There are endless possibilities. Here are some; staff timekeeping, 'over the counter' sales for a particular product or range of products, reducing complaints, reducing debtors, increasing booster vaccinations as a percentage of reminders, improved control of waste and so on.

Consider offering a bonus to support staff who spot charges which have been forgotten by the consulting veterinarian. Another approach is to distribute to the staff a percentage (possibly 10%) of practice growth in real terms (excluding the impact of inflation) over the same period during the previous year. Do not forget the possibility too, of deducting sums from your staff salaries for some particularly heinous 'crime'. How about a fine of £10 every time you hear a member of staff apologising about your fees?

However generous the financial package may be, you can be sure that it alone will not motivate your staff. All motivation, it is said, is self motivation. The secret is to stimulate and encourage self worth, self esteem and self motivation. Self esteem will be generated by achievement, recognised by self and by others. Perhaps the secret of motivating staff is to help them to set themselves tough targets, measure the results, recognise their achievements and praise the results.

Some take the view that incentive arrangements simply result in employees receiving salary levels which they should have been entitled to in the first place. Some employees resent the suggestion that

there is any need to use financial bait to encourage them to carry out the job for which they have been employed and trained.

The most difficult approach to incentive payments for support or professional staff is for them to be based on net profit. As we have argued elsewhere, profit is merely an opinion. It would be necessary at the outset to determine and agree with the employee and then document precisely how gross income and all costs are determined. It is necessary to accept that all practice financial data may be exposed to employee's scrutiny and we believe that the calculation of an employee's monthly salary based on an opinion is destined to create major problems sooner or later.

While the range of possible incentive schemes is limited only by the creative imagination of the practice leadership, the end result so often is to pay a base salary and incentive payment which is close to what the employee was worth in the first place. The attraction of incentive arrangements for the practice owner is that the management responsibility to determine an appropriate salary level is replaced by the mechanics of the system. In our experience, most incentive arrangements do not have a long lasting effect in practice. They do provide a shot in the arm, a short term stimulus but sooner or later employees become disillusioned with the system and if it is to be retained, it must be constantly upgraded and revamped.

One of the main reasons why incentive programmes do not work especially well for support staff is that professional services, not product sales, are the primary focus in practice. Ethical standards demand that veterinarians and their staff should be blind to the economic gain of service in favour of the well-being of the patient. The procedure which achieves the highest level of gross revenue may not yield the most appropriate medical result. We accept that the vast majority of employees do maintain their own personal ethic for service and conduct but recognise that one or two greedy individuals could devastate the practice reputation by enlightened self interest. Clients are much wiser than we sometimes believe. They will very soon recognise that they are being handled by an incentive hungry member of staff.

Their Prime Role

How would you define the primary role of your staff? How about 'to acquire and keep clients for the practice'. Would that be a stimulating topic of discussion for your next practice meeting?

We are sure that the majority of veterinary practice staff are willing and able to be used much more productively than their bosses anticipate. Talk to them, use them, involve them. Discuss your draft mission statement with them. Ask them to help you to identify day to day problems and take note of their proposals for solving them. Remember that all employees deserve basic human decency and kindness. Your staff will respect you more as a leader if you can offer them a little care and a lot of thoughtfulness. Courtesy and good manners are an essential component of effective personnel management. Your employees seek:

- APPRECIATION; Tell them how much you appreciate their hard work and enthusiasm. Drop them a note from time to time; remember birthdays; ask about their hopes and their anxieties, their achievements and their support. Say 'thank you' and mean it.
- RECOGNITION; Introduce them to your clients, include them in a staff directory, include their picture and a 'thumb-nail sketch' about them in your practice brochure. Promote them in your newsletter and maybe provide them with their own business cards.
- SOCIAL NEEDS; Your staff will only enjoy their work if they also enjoy a happy working relationship with the other staff members. Do all you can to encourage a warm and friendly staff atmosphere. Provide a staff lounge area, coffee facilities or even a microwave oven. Encourage them to decorate their room and the public parts of the practice at Christmas so that they can work and play together and have some fun.

Don't overdo it! Don't become over-familiar with your staff and don't let them become over-familiar with you. You must maintain a position of being able to make unbiased, detached judgements about their contribution to the success of the practice.

- INVOLVEMENT; Seek the advice of the practice support staff, informally and formally at staff meetings. Involve them in brainstorming sessions. Seek their opinion about those things which could be done better and ask them how.

Equitable Pay for Partners

Veterinary practice owners throughout the world understand more than anyone the degree to which taxation picks their pockets. Government constantly moves the goal posts and professional advice will always be necessary to deal with the continuous changes in revenue and capital taxation.

The common goal of seeking to preserve capital has resulted in a worldwide tendency for veterinarians to postpone their retirement as clinicians. As they grow older they have a dual need for more free time which must be balanced with the economic need to maintain the standard of living to which they have become accustomed. In many practices therefore senior partners want to continue to be involved in the practice but not with the same intensity as they had in their younger years. It becomes necessary then to establish equitable pay arrangements among partners which recognise the level of their investment on the one hand, and the different amount of time they are able or wish to commit to the practice on the other. Younger partners, often with children who have yet to be educated, clothed, fed and nurtured will generally be interested in working longer and harder in order to afford the life style they choose. More experienced partners, on the other hand, no longer have as many financial pressures and will often elect to receive a lower level of remuneration for the time they allocate to practice business in order to enjoy an enhanced quality of life.

The question then is how best to establish an equitable, fair and clear system for paying partners which recognises the varying levels of their input. We often hear senior partners at meetings and conferences boast that money is not really an important factor in their professional relationships. However, just let one partner's income fall short of what he has been used to and watch the fall-out in a disgruntled group. To another more financially secure partner, cash beomes less of an incentive as family commitments wane. On the other hand, even when individuals have an adequate level of savings for their retirement, the fear of un-anticipated costs in years to come causes even the most balanced and realistically forward looking veterinarian to fear the possibility of not being in a position of functioning independently without the assistance of family, friends and government.

The first step then is to make sure that all parties are talking about the same definition of 'fair and equitable'. Equitable is not the same as equal. Equitable implies a *pro rata* share of practice profit based upon relative contributions of both time and money.

Although the options available for structuring an equitable compensation package for partners are as varied as the partners themselves, there are some basic premises that need to be considered by the partners in dividing the available profits. Most practices will recognise three distinct factors which must be considered;

- The amount of time spent as a clinician.
- A return based on the level of equity investment.
- The level of contribution for management, leadership and other duties designed to enhance practice performance.

The first two of these elements are easy to deal with. The first tranche of profit must be used to pay partners for the time they invest as clinicians in the practice. The interests of the partner as an 'employee' must be respected and protected before that of an equity owner. The risks of ownership may not be rewarded until the costs of all the employees have been met.

The third element to be considered is the contribution that each partner makes in the area of management, practice development, personnel or any other essential but non-clinical activity which is perceived to be essential to practice success.

This is the most difficult element to define or to measure. Its significance will be determined by the view taken by the partners about the significance and value of leadership and management in achieving practice success. For example, a practice in which the principal or partners believe that clinical work is the only meaningful measure of activity, will place little emphasis on management or contributory leadership. Here, the third element of reward is likely to be simply based on the number of transactions, gross income or average transaction value per veterinarian.

Another practice may take the view that the first tier of compensation as a clinician more than compensates the partners for their productive capability but wishes to reward partners in addition on the basis of their availability. In that situation, the hours spent by each individual partner in the conduct of the practice, however that time is spent, will be calculated and monitored. The partners may consider that time spent in the furtherance of the practice interest will have a value whether or not it contributes directly to practice revenue. Others may recognise the importance of setting aside time for management but believe that 'management' time is only worth a proportion of 'clinical' time.

It will be a matter then for the partners alone, or in discussion with their accountant or management consultant, to determine any 'fair and equitable' system which will enable them to fulfil their objectives. Reference to the practice mission statement may assist them in assessing what factors are truly important in the practice and help them to clarify their view about the value of 'management' time.

Developing the Key Practice Manager

To our knowledge there are no schools of veterinary practice management which have as yet graduated classes although a number of colleges in the United States are planning to establish such courses.

In the United States, the Veterinary Hospital Managers' Association and the American Animal Hospital Association are developing areas of knowledge for practice managers to develop a basic skill. During the last ten years, the Veterinary Hospital Managers' Association has mounted a number of seminars for practice managers at their annual and regional meetings. The American Animal Hospital Association has been amongst the forerunners of those developing practice management concepts. The focus has to date been directed more towards hospital directors and member veterinarians but in recent years, the Association has focused more on the needs of practice managers. A seminar for practice managers is now scheduled in September of every year at Las Vegas, Nevada.

Veterinary practice managers require a wide range of management skills as well as a thorough knowledge of veterinary practice. They need to understand the business of veterinary practice,

i.e., the diagnostic, prophylactic, medical, surgical and other services which the practice provides. At the same time, they must be skilled in all the management disciplines and have a particular perception of veterinary practice as a business.

We believe that more and more veterinary practices will see the need to separate the roles of the equity owner, clinicians and business manager and to allocate the appropriate area of responsibility to individuals with the knowledge and skills to carry them out. The practice manager's responsibility is to become the head, heart, and soul of the financial and operational management of the practice.

7

Financial Management

Financial Management

Measuring Practice Success

Many measures could be used to monitor the success of your practice. Here are some:

- Quality of professional care and attention for clients and patients.
- Degree of client satisfaction.
- Maintenance of patient health.
- Quality of clinical records.
- A sound financial performance.
- The level of salaries and conditions of work for all staff members.
- Required return on the owner's investment in the practice.
- Good reputation and respect for clients, patients and staff.
- Practice image of which the owners and all concerned are proud.

Most practice principals are able to make some subjective judgments about each of these factors, but many of them are difficult to measure objectively. Sooner or later, the success of the practice will have to be measured financially. Tax inspectors (agents), bank managers, accountants, prospective incoming partners or purchasers will all wish to be satisfied that, in addition to all the other subjective measures, here is a veterinary business which is financially sound.

A Successful, Viable and Profitable Business

If you want to continue to enjoy your career in veterinary practice, you surely want to be part of a successful, viable and profitable business. While recognising that money isn't everything and that practice success can be measured in a variety of ways, the common measure of performance is

a financial one. Continuing financial success in veterinary practice depends on a commitment to quality professional service.

The Financial Plan

The definition of management which incorporates planning, organisation and control functions can be used to provide a framework for considering financial matters. Planning can be likened to preparing a route from a particular starting point to a chosen destination. In financial planning, therefore, the first and crucially important task, is to identify precisely where you are now and how you got there. In other words, prepare a financial statement for the practice which identifies the current financial position. It should summarise financial performance over the previous three years for example, and identify the practice's financial strengths and weaknesses.

For the moment, let us consider a broad approach to an examination of practice financial strengths and weaknesses. Some value judgements need to be made about some or all of the following parameters:

- Gross revenue trends in recent years.
- Practice growth in real terms (bearing in mind the impact of inflation).
- Profit trends.
- Cash flow.
- Case volume trends.
- The level and significance of each of the practice costs.
- Liquidity.
- Debtor level.
- Stock turnover.
- Gearing.

Now you have some indication of your present position in financial terms. You will need to decide what specific financial objectives to set over the period of the plan to calculate the level of income needed. Also you will need to estimate the costs of achieving that income. Profit is simply the difference between the level of income earned and the costs incurred in earning it over a particular period of time.

Up to now you may have assumed that practice profits are largely the result of influences beyond your control. Perhaps your practice deals with all the work that presents itself. You note with some interest at your financial year end, the costs incurred and you express satisfaction or dismay at the profit level you achieved.

Take Control

Now, however, we are talking about setting a financial strategy in which you take control of what happens in the practice.

STEP 1: — Decide what profit figure you intend to achieve each year in your two year strategy. Be bold, be specific and write it down.

STEP 2: — Examine the practice costs from last year. Rethink every single cost item and identify the property, equipment and personnel resources likely to be needed over the period. Identify the fixed and variable costs of those resources in financial terms or as a proportion of practice turnover.

STEP 3: — Calculate what level of revenue the practice will need to generate to finance those costs and achieve a predetermined surplus profit level.

Remember that practice revenue is simply a function of the number of clients who come through your doors and the average sum they spend on your services. A number of possible options for increasing practice turnover and improving the quality of service to clients could be achieved. Consider these thoughts:

You could;

- increase case volume.
- increase the professional fee, in real terms, for each service item.
- increase your charges for items sold, dispensed or utilised in providing those services.

- where appropriate increase the number of services provided or goods supplied per transaction.

Each of these last three measures will result in an increased average transaction value. We strongly advise that your practice should monitor case volume and average transaction value on a regular basis. The simplest approach is to regard each chargeable invoice as one unit of volume.

An important part of the financial plan will then be concerned with precisely how the practice intends to generate the target income level and what trends can be anticipated for case volume, fees and average transaction values.

Financial Projections

A strategic financial plan should include projected profit and loss statements for each of the next two years and a detailed budget for the first year with a monthly cashflow statement.

However carefully planned, the projections can only give a broad indication of what is expected to happen in the future. It would be wise to give an indication in your plan of the best possible scenario, the worst and an estimate of the likeliest outcome.

Cash Flow Statement

A major benefit of preparing cash flow statements regularly is that it will enable the practice to keep the bank manager appraised of progress. Experience suggests that bank managers are generally positive and helpful but don't like unpleasant surprises. Always try to work on the basis of keeping one step ahead. Cash flow forecasting will enable the practice owner to notify the bank two or three months ahead if significant changes in overdraft or other requirements are anticipated.

The statement should incorporate any assumptions made and indicate the positive steps to be taken to ensure that revenue targets are achieved.

The financial plan also needs to take into account any significant capital expenditure over the period with an outline timetable, method of payment, likely costs and an indication of the additional income expected as a result of the investment.

Finally, it will need to include a review of the funding of the practice and incorporate a brief indication of likely balance sheet values for each of the two years ahead.

Practice Accounts

You will need to consider the two quite separate but important sources of information relating to the financial performance of the practice.

Financial Accounts

Financial accounts are prepared annually, usually by the practice accountant. They are required for statutory and other purposes and are primarily used by third parties like bank managers, statutory bodies and government agencies and by potential partners and purchasers. The information which the financial accounts contain is of limited value for practice management purposes, largely because much of the data from which they are derived is many months out of date.

Management Accounts

Management accounts, on the other hand, are prepared for internal use only. They are designed by the practice owner or manager with the assistance and advice of the practice accountant or other financial advisers. They incorporate only those items of information which are required to monitor practice performance and are used to identify adverse trends at an early stage. This ensures that appropriate corrective measures can be taken. This is the control aspect referred to in the above definition of management.

Management accounts are regarded as a tool for effective decision making. Financial and other data are collected to provide managers with the information they need, at the time and in the form they want. Here are some suggestions for the financial and other quantitative information useful to manage a practice. Identify sources of revenue by:
  SERVICE such as:

small animal consultations
small animal house calls
small animal surgical / in-patient work
small animal treatments
small animal medication
radiography and other diagnostic work
large animal / equine consultations
large animal surgical / procedures and diagnostic work
large animal medication
'over the counter' and other merchandising sales

PREMISES such as
  main hospital
  practice branch
  satellite clinics

EMPLOYEES such as
  consulting veterinarian
  technician / veterinary nurse

PATIENT SPECIES such as
  dogs
  cats
  horses
  cattle
  sheep
  pigs
  poultry
  exotic species

COSTS.
Identify items of expenditure using a limited number of specific cost headings e.g:

- Drugs and other stock items
- Food and accessories
- Other animal health products
- Professional salaries and allied costs
- Other staff salaries and allied costs
- Property rates, taxes and insurance
- Heat/light/power
- Telephone/stationery
- Repairs/renewals
- Motor/travel
- Legal/accountancy
- Finance costs
- Miscellaneous

The American Animal Hospital Association has published a comprehensive Chart of Accounts

REVENUE ANALYSIS AS AT END DECEMBER 1992 (All data Ex VAT)						
Last year			Jan 91	Feb 91	Mar 91	Apr 91
RPI			130.2	130.9	131.4	133.1
Turnover last year		197154.36	13507.09	10186.22	11684.74	15775.33
Case volume last year		15563	1156	867	949	1174
This year			Jan 92	Feb 92	Mar 92	Apr 92
RPI			135.6	136.3	136.7	138.8
Staff available		Average				
Principals/partners		1.67	1.00	1.75	2.00	1.00
Employed V.S. FTE		0.08	0.00	0.00	0.00	0.00
Total V.S. in month		1.75	1.00	1.75	2.00	1.00
Other staff FTE		2.25	2.00	2.00	1.50	2.50
Ratio other: V.S.		1.38	2.00	1.14	0.75	2.50
Revenue	Revenue %	Turnover				
Services	68.38	141597.87	13017.84	9727.41	12369.91	9553.34
Medication	21.78	45098.65	2542.20	2874.23	4065.08	3763.48
Miscellaneous	9.84	20374.16	1842.42	1174.98	1340.99	1072.46
Turnover this year	100.00	207070.68	17402.46	13776.62	17775.98	14389.28
Change in turnover		9.55%	28.84%	35.25%	52.13%	-8.79%
RPI adjusted change		5.60%	23.71%	29.89%	46.23%	-12.53%
MAT turnover this year		197154.36	201049.73	204640.13	210731.37	209345.32
Case volume this year		15622	1175	1155	1414	1172
MAT case volume		15563	15582	15870	16335	16333
Change in case volume		3.84%	1.64%	33.22%	49.00%	-0.17%
Statistics						
Revenue per V.S.		10517.90	17402.46	7872.35	8887.99	14389.28
Case vol. per V.S.		794.81	1175.00	660.00	707.00	1172.00
Medication:services ratio		0.32	0.20	0.30	0.33	0.39
Average transaction fee		13.34	14.81	11.93	12.57	12.28

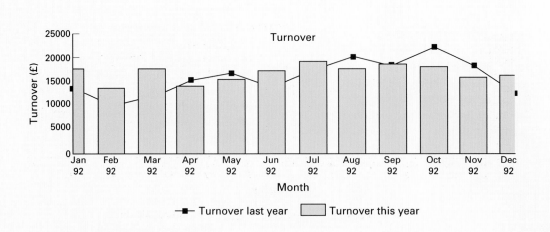

REVENUE ANALYSIS AS AT END DECEMBER 1992 (All data Ex VAT)							
May 91	**Jun 91**	**Jul 91**	**Aug 91**	**Sep 91**	**Oct 91**	**Nov 91**	**Dec 91**
133.5	134.1	133.8	134.1	134.6	135.1	135.6	135.7
17079.54	14199.03	18113.05	20945.47	19284.96	23231.40	19425.21	13722.32
1337	1104	1619	1759	1613	1518	1380	1087

May 92	**Jun 92**	**Jul 92**	**Aug 92**	**Sep 92**	**Oct 92**	**Nov 92**	**Dec 92**
139.3	139.3	138.8	138.9	139.4	139.9	139.7	139.2
2.00	1.75	2.00	1.50	1.50	2.00	2.00	1.50
0.00	0.00	0.00	0.00	0.00	0.00	0.00	1.00
2.00	1.75	2.00	1.50	1.50	2.00	2.00	2.50
2.50	2.00	2.50	2.50	2.50	2.00	2.50	2.50
1.25	1.14	1.25	1.67	1.67	1.00	1.25	1.00
10847.70	13393.99	12957.27	11494.41	12955.12	12621.79	10287.22	12371.87
3000.36	2887.75	4486.19	4982.77	4485.79	4056.38	4746.56	3207.86
1779.28	1401.78	2292.36	1754.55	2006.51	2061.00	1793.43	1854.40
15627.34	17683.52	19735.82	18231.73	19447.42	18739.17	16827.21	17434.13
-8.50%	24.54%	8.96%	-12.96%	0.84%	-19.34%	-13.37%	27.05%
-12.31%	19.89%	5.03%	-15.96%	-2.63%	-22.10%	-15.92%	23.85%
207893.12	211377.61	213000.38	210286.64	210449.10	205956.87	203358.87	207070.68
978	1348	1517	1534	1429	1428	1219	1218
15974	16254	16152	15927	15742	15652	15491	15622
-26.85%	25.36%	-6.30%	-12.79%	-11.47%	-5.93%	-11.67%	12.05%
7813.67	10104.87	9867.91	12154.49	12964.95	9369.59	8413.61	6973.65
489.00	790.86	758.50	1022.67	952.00	714.00	609.50	487.20
0.28	0.22	0.35	0.43	0.35	0.32	0.46	0.26
15.98	12.78	13.01	11.89	13.62	13.12	13.80	14.31

FIG. 1 Management accounting information used by a number of practices in the UK.

PERFORMANCE AND COST ANALYSIS AS AT END DECEMBER 1992 (All data Ex VAT)					
This year		**Y.T.D.**	**Jan 92**	**Feb 92**	**Mar 92**	**Apr 92**
Expected productive hours per veterinary surgeon per month				100 hours		
Hourly professional charge			53.22	53.22	53.22	53.22
Total service hours		215.66	244.60	182.78	232.43	179.51
Hours per V.S.		132.40	244.60	104.44	116.21	179.51
Costs analysis	Turnover %	Average				
Drugs	26.08%	4500.17	3515.51	4478.15	2964.82	5895.63
Prof. salaries	0.89%	152.78	0.00	0.00	0.00	0.00
Support salaries	15.18%	2618.95	1337.96	1806.85	2957.76	837.09
Rent/rates/ins.	2.93%	506.02	571.00	0.00	98.62	443.32
Consultancy	0.41%	71.07	0.00	0.00	852.80	0.00
Heat/power	1.19%	204.99	229.87	0.00	896.53	26.27
Tel./stationary	4.71%	812.70	930.80	1321.93	112.49	499.45
Rep./renewals	4.44%	765.52	829.82	8.00	2367.57	149.91
Motor	6.49%	1120.19	221.54	905.80	3732.70	723.98
Legal/Acc't.	1.02%	176.61	350.00	557.37	0.00	150.00
Finance costs	8.01%	1382.34	0.00	2172.99	2494.72	1022.25
Miscellaneous	5.46%	941.42	1144.18	1202.92	1260.66	585.53
Total	76.80%	13252.74	9130.68	12454.01	17738.67	10333.43
Average gross profit		**4003.15**	**8271.78**	**1322.61**	**37.31**	**4055.85**
Profit as percentage of turnover		**23.20%**	**47.53%**	**9.60%**	**0.21%**	**28.19%**

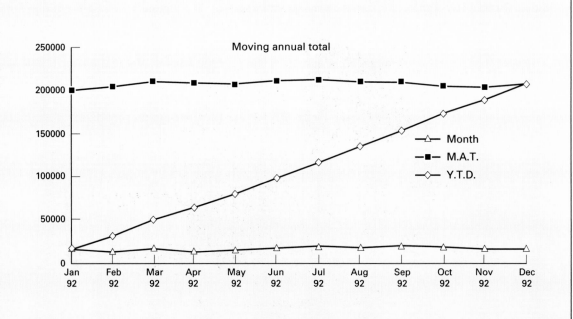

PERFORMANCE AND COST ANALYSIS AS AT END DECEMBER 1992							
May 92	Jun 92	Jul 92	Aug 92	Sep 92	Oct 92	Nov 92	Dec 92
Vet FTEs in 12 months to date: 2.16							
53.22	53.46	53.46	53.46	57.60	57.66	57.66	57.66
203.83	250.54	242.37	215.01	224.92	218.90	178.41	214.57
101.91	143.17	121.19	143.34	149.94	109.45	89.21	85.83
3118.45	5269.77	5741.95	4494.78	4802.74	5112.61	4220.86	4386.71
0.00	0.00	0.00	0.00	0.00	0.00	0.00	1833.33
2310.89	1333.39	5905.05	1507.31	2565.45	3328.85	3525.47	4011.28
234.00	194.92	1850.00	234.00	234.00	639.34	970.66	602.33
0.00	0.00	0.00	0.00	0.00	0.00	0.00	0.00
0.00	610.61	0.00	0.00	292.60	0.00	0.00	403.95
1041.09	331.00	524.20	1092.52	1552.40	1084.73	986.70	275.07
10.40	843.24	590.02	3359.09	551.65	25.60	402.78	48.12
571.19	1496.71	468.00	1450.23	1018.39	493.62	736.90	1623.21
0.00	7.00	200.00	0.00	660.00	150.00	45.00	0.00
431.68	1655.30	0.00	1492.28	2661.10	526.94	1311.39	2819.42
660.99	863.03	623.10	675.86	1384.90	342.71	1493.00	1060.18
8378.69	12604.97	15902.32	14306.07	15723.23	11704.40	13692.76	17063.60
7248.65	5078.55	3833.50	3925.66	3724.19	7034.77	3134.45	370.53
46.38%	28.72%	19.42%	21.53%	19.15%	37.54%	18.63%	2.13%

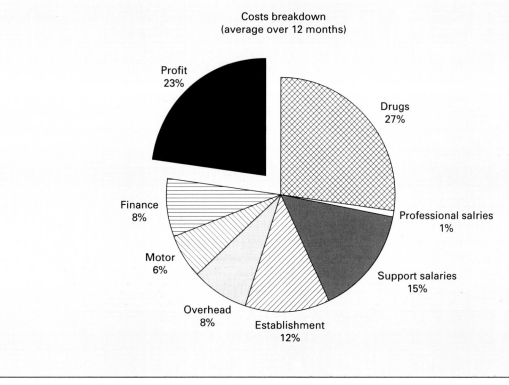

Costs breakdown
(average over 12 months)

Profit 23%
Drugs 27%
Professional salries 1%
Support salaries 15%
Establishment 12%
Overhead 8%
Motor 6%
Finance 8%

FIG. 2 Management accounting information used by a number of practices in the UK.

which is used by an increasing number of veterinarians and their accountants. It is important to select the simplest breakdown of income and expenditure to accommodate the needs of individual practices and their advisers.

Management Reports

The Reporting Process

Having accumulated the necessary data, the next major question to consider is how best to utilise it to prepare reports in a form which will be of practical value for management purposes.

The process of selecting a computer based system for veterinary practice starts with an evaluation of detailed practice requirements which is then converted into a specification for a system appropriate for that practice. The same approach is taken in planning a management reporting system. The requirements of the practice manager and the practice owner may, however, not be the same. The practice manager for instance, may consider the production of management accounting reports as the end product of the system, while the owner/director will regard the management reports simply as the tools to be used to monitor performance. It will also indicate the need for management action to correct adverse trends or other problems which may be revealed.

It may be that the practice manager and the practice owner are the same individual. If not, it is most important that the requirements of each are clarified before the layout of management reports is finalised. There have been a number of instances in which the value of an expensive data recording and retrieval system has been put in jeopardy because the practice owner is unaware of what the manager is doing. The manager, on the other hand, regards the system as all important and cannot appreciate that it only exists to monitor performance and to indicate where and when corrective or other management action is required.

Included in this book are typical management accounting layouts (Figures 1 and 2). They are illustrations of the sort of data which can be prepared on a standard spreadsheet and printed on one sheet of paper. Yet they demonstrate

trends for a number of parameters over a two year period. Two or more heads may be better than one in planning such layouts. We recommend a brain-storming session in which the practice owner, the manager and the practice accountant are involved in determining the details of the required management reports, their production frequency and the individuals who should receive them.

Discussion with the practice accountant is also necessary to clarify what information is required for;

- the annual financial accounts, prepared in accordance with generally accepted accounting principles for statutory and other purposes
- management accounts which are prepared for internal management purposes only.

Comparative Data

A major advantage of regular, accurate management accounting data is to enable management to draw valid comparisons between individual employees or groups of employees, premises or services or to compare performance with previous periods. Effective budgeting must be based on accurate historical information and involve close monitoring of performance to identify adverse or other trends and variances from budget. Early recognition of such trends and decision making designed to correct them are the essence of sound management.

Management accounting information can also be used to draw comparisons between the practice and similar practices. No two veterinary practices are the same. Their objectives may differ, the resources available to them and the market in which they operate may be very different. Comparative data may still be valid but it is important to understand that statistical or other information for a particular practice relates only to the circumstances for that practice. Measures and trends may be neither better nor worse for that practice than for any other, but simply different. Comparisons should be used for intelligent assessment not mindless compliance. The important point is to spot differences, ask yourself why they occur, what they mean and whether lessons can be learned as a result.

Analysis

Management accounting involves the retrieval of data for management purposes and the recognition of changes and trends in practice performance. However, if the trend is not explained and no action is taken, there is little point in going to the expense and trouble of collecting the information in the first place. Analysis demands that variations from budget or adverse trends are explained. Why has this happened and what can we do about it? You will need to explain performance fluctuations and determine whether the problem relates to delivery of service, personnel or to some change in market needs or perceptions. Are you the cause of an issue or does the problem lie with your colleagues, partners or staff? Performance ratios may be valuable and you should specifically examine individual cost and revenue relationships to gross income.

Professional salary costs are a good example. A number of practices employing several veterinarians utilise a number of individual performance based measures for determining individual salaries. An analysis of gross income generated by each veterinarian is one measure, but one which does not take into account the profit resulting from those efforts. Identifying the individuals contribution to practice profit may or may not be possible but there are a number of other measures which may measure the individuals contribution to practice success more fairly. They may include for example, the number of new clients attracted to the practice, productive hours worked per month, the individuals contribution to the in-house continuing education of staff members and a number of other measures. Also monitor the contribution to profits made by each consulting room, the laboratory, the treatment room and any other area in the practice. Take into consideration the number of hours each room is used productively to generate revenue. Should you expand the hours you are open? Look at the figures every day. Keep asking how performance can be improved. How can staff, equipment and facilities be more effectively, economically or efficiently used to improve the service to clients and the profit margin for the business?

In planning monthly management reports for your practice, you, the practice manager or your colleagues will need to develop a routine for considering the implications of the information and any required corrective measures. Management accounting reports should include some or all of the following information:

- revenue 'this month' and each month last year
- revenue this month and each month to date this year
- revenue analysis by service and by veterinarian
- case volume 'this month' and each month last year
- case volume this month and each month to date this year
- moving annual total case volume
- moving annual total revenue
- average transaction value
- medication/service ratio

The Need for Discipline

The effective use of management accounts requires a measure of discipline:

- to identify the data required
- to establish a manual or computer based system to collect the data regularly, preferably monthly
- to study and interpret the results, to identify adverse trends and to take immediate steps to correct them.

Management accounting requires planning discipline but at the same time must be simple and easy to understand. If you try to set up anything too complex, the data simply will not be used and will be filed away 'for future reference' i.e. never.

It is the task of the appropriate clerical or administrative staff to ensure that the data retrieval system works effectively and efficiently. The management role is not concerned with the regular collection of the data but with identifying what is required, the design of a system to collect it and its use for management purposes.

The data need not be 100% accurate as long as the same basis is used to collect or calculate the information on a regular basis. This ensures that trends or other changes can be identified quickly.

The Need to Plan

Our impression is that in most practices, systems have been established over the years which do an excellent job in recording information and a reasonable job in reporting it. The big problem appears to be that veterinarians do not allocate the time or resources to compare, analyse and plan. Planning in particular is the crucial element of management which seems to be missing in many practices and planning requires a vision of the future. A vision which can only be determined by sound leadership and the preparation of a mission statement which summarises practice objectives and shared values for service in the community.

The Prime Financial Objective

The prime financial objective of any business enterprise is to survive. Books on cost and management accounting demonstrate the use of a large number of possible financial measures and ratios. Business survival depends on maintaining a healthy balance between PROFIT, CASH and GEARING. Consider each of these in turn.

Cash

Cash is real, cash is a fact. There can be no argument about it. You have got it or you haven't. Cash or sufficient credit is needed to pay staff and all the regular bills. The practice's strength in respect of cash is called its LIQUIDITY. A number of liquidity measures can be used but two are most common.

Working Capital

The relationship between current assets (stock, debtors, bank balances and cash) and current liabilities (creditors, overdraft and short term loans) represents the working capital. Clearly a healthy balance between the two with the value of current assets at or greater than the value of

current liabilities will ensure that the practice is unlikely to be faced with demands for cash which it is unable to meet.

Acid Test

This ratio is a much more stringent test of an organisation's ability to meet short term commitments. Stock (inventory) is not included in the ratio as it cannot be converted into cash very quickly.

Remember, businesses can be highly profitable and yet run out of cash. On the other hand they may be cash rich (in the short term) and yet be unprofitable. In the short term a business can survive without profit as long as it has adequate cash resources but it can't survive without cash even if it is making substantial profits. It is crucial to appreciate the difference between cash and profitability and to monitor them both.

A major part of your business plan will be to identify and monitor the flow of receipts and payments so that you:

- have enough cash to meet liabilities when due.
- monitor actual cash flow against plan and if necessary, adjust the priorities.
- see the effect of planned capital investment on cashflow and liquidity.
- can discuss trends in advance with your financial advisers and with your bank.

Profit

Profit is merely an OPINION and is a measure of the change in value of the enterprise at the end of the period compared with its value at the beginning. An increase implies a profit while a decrease implies a loss.

Profit is a misused and grossly misunderstood term. Profit has alternative meanings dependent upon the type of business organisation structure and on the specific tax laws appropriate to the country where the business operates. Even generally accepted accounting principles differ from country to country in terms of what profit should mean. For the purposes of this book and to initiate a discussion about a standard starting point within the veterinary profession world-wide we suggest the following definition of profit:

Profit is the difference between the revenue generated (not the same as the income received) during a period and the costs involved, without regard to a return on investment for the equity of the business, in generating that revenue.

The revenue generated is equivalent to the total of fees earned, not the total cash received. In many practices cash received and fee income generated approximate each other. As practices grow there will normally be a disparity between fees earned and cash collected as the young practice is building up its working capital in the form of debtors (receivables). As the practice continues to mature, the rate of increase in debtors slows down until actual fees earned and cash received approximate one another.

Proceeds from borrowings or payments of accounts outstanding are not sources of fee income and do not affect profit. Similarly repayments of principal on sums borrowed is not an expenditure that reduces profit.

Expenditure on items of a capital nature are not true costs of operation nor are they expenses that would reduce profit. For example, the purchase of equipment, furniture and fixtures, increases in drug stocks (inventory), purchase of practice vehicles or investments made for leasehold improvements will not affect profit. Although profit is not affected by capital expenditure, the reduction in value of capital items over a period of time is regarded as a deduction from profits. There are various conventions for reducing the value of fixed assets dependent on the veterinarians country of residence. These accepted accounting principles have an impact on the individuals tax liabilities. In some countries it is not uncommon to have four or more different depreciation conventions calculated for one component asset and recorded in a number of different ways. In the United States, for example, one depreciation calculation is made to conform to generally accepted accounting principles, another is used to calculate Federal Income Tax liability, another would be to calculate the alternative minimum tax liability, another is used to calculate the adjusted current earnings for the business and finally, there is the possibility of a separate

state calculation for income tax purposes. To compound matters further, in countries such as the United States, there is a secondary source of taxing for personal property tax and a separate depreciation reduction is calculated for tangible personal property at the state or county level.

The ideal situation from the veterinarians point of view is one in which management has an opportunity to establish a sinking fund to replace the asset due to wear, tear and obsolescence i.e to save for the future, rather than to respond to the historical recovery of past expenditure. As a result, managers might recognise more easily that funds must be set aside to create a fund to replace the asset. Calculation of the size of the fund must be based upon the current replacement value of the asset and not its historical cost, net book value or actual cash value. For example, if a bank of cages cost US$1,000 three years ago, and $1,400 today, the economic decline in the value of the asset would be based on a ten-year useful life on a straight-line method. This means that 10% of the fair market value, or US$140 ($1,400 x 10%) would be the amount held as the sinking fund provision.

This is a derivation of the generally accepted accounting principles in most countries but also takes into consideration the replenishment cost of an asset which is a more critical issue for practising veterinarians. Financial statements submitted to banks, tax returns prepared for governmental entities and other financial and valuation reports, may not take into consideration the issue of the economic decline in the value of an asset as a provision based on replacement cost. However, veterinarians who should be constantly aware of the need to replenish assets to provide the highest level of veterinary care, must be concerned about the availability of adequate funds to pay for them.

Some countries have already adopted this idea of replacement cost value. The accounting literature is littered with debates between accountants in various countries on the validity of reflecting a reduction in net profit for replacement cost. Our thoughts are not intended to add more confusion to the issue, but merely to remind veterinarians that a major management task in practice is to plan for the replacement of equipment in an increasingly competitive market with growing requirements for technical and other capital investment.

What is left over, after taking into consideration income earned and expenses incurred including provision for the economic decline in the value of assets, is an appropriately managed level of profit.

In a sole trader or partnership situation the owner's or partner's personal tax liabilities are based on the so called 'profit' of the enterprise. Clearly an assessment of the financial performance of an enterprise must take into account all the legitimate costs involved including the 'salary' of the practice principal. For management purposes veterinary practice owners should consider themselves as employees. They are entitled to earn a fair salary for their clinical services rendered. Their role as managers must be regarded as an additional cost to the practice while the resultant true profit will reflect their return on investment.

Profit implies growth but if the level of profit is merely an expression of opinion by the practice principal and accountants some decision will need to be made as to whether one should aim for a large profit or a small one. For tax purposes the smaller the profit the less tax you will have to pay, subject to the approval of your accounts by the tax inspectorate. On the other hand if you plan to sell the practice or a share of it or if you seek to raise cash or impress third parties you will wish to maximise practice growth/performance as measured by profit.

Gearing

Gearing measures the amount of OPM (other people's money) as a proportion of the total finance invested in the practice. If there are no bank borrowings or other liabilities and the practice is owned solely by the practice principal, there would be no gearing. While it is recognised that the balance sheet valuation of fixed assets often fails to reflect a realistic current valuation of the practice property, gearing is frequently measured by comparing total liabilities with total assets on balance sheet valuations. There is nothing wrong with borrowing for business purposes. The simplest test of whether significant

borrowing is justified is to ask whether the profit which can be achieved as a result of the borrowing is greater that the cost of incurring the debt. If you can make a return of 15% on money borrowed at 10% that's fine. If you only achieve 8% on the same money for any length of time, perhaps you should think again.

It is crucial to monitor LIQUIDITY, PROFITABILITY and GEARING if nothing else. If any one of them goes wrong it will have an immediate impact on the others. Any practice must develop a strategy for managing all three.

Two other financial measures or ratios can be of considerable value in monitoring practice performance:

Stock Control

A significant proportion of practice income is derived from the purchase and sale of goods. A practice houses a stock of drugs, disposable and sundry items, some of which will be used by the veterinarians and staff in the day to day running of the practice. Some will be sold or dispensed to clients. Since the holding of stock ties up cash and increases the amount of capital employed, it should be the aim to keep stock levels to a minimum compatible with providing an adequate level of service to clients.

The profitability of the stock keeping function will depend on two factors:

The Margin

While there may be legal, ethical and marketing pressures to restrict margins for particular products or group of products, be advised to work on the basis of a minimum margin of 50% of the selling price (i.e., markup of 100% of cost price).

Stock Turnover

Stock turnover is the number of times stock holding is turned over per annum. The figure is calculated from the cost of stock (profit and loss figure) divided by the value of stock at balance sheet valuation. Many small animal practices, for example, would aim to rotate stock at least ten times per annum.

The ideal stock level is one in which key drug stock items never run out. This ensures a good level of service for clients while minimising practice costs and maximising profits.

The question is how much stock should be ordered and what level of stock should be held. There is no easy answer and the appropriate stock level may be different for each individual product. What is important is to recognise that the costs of maintaining an adequate level of stock includes:

- The cost of purchase per unit.
- The ordering cost. The time involved in determining the need to restock and to place the order; the running costs of the internal control methods for checking delivery notes and invoices; unpacking, shelving and monitoring items 'to follow'.
- The cost of holding the stock including the opportunity cost (the cost that could have been saved by investing the money in a safe investment elsewhere) and other holding costs such as staff time, the cost of shelf space, breakages, losses and an appropriate share of overhead costs.

It has been estimated that the ordering, holding and opportunity costs may be as high as 20% to 25% of the total annual cost of stock. Practice owners and managers would do well to keep this figure in mind in determining stock levels, markup and the required margin. A veterinary practice, for example, which operated on the basis of marking up overall stock prices by 50% ie to achieve a gross margin of 33%, would discover by a close examination of all the appropriate costs that the profit level achieved was much smaller than anticipated.

Credit Control

Debtor turnover is a measure of the practice's credit control and can also have a significant effect on working capital requirements. Most small animal practices aim for a turnover figure significantly less than 7 days while large animal and equine practices would not be surprised at figures well in excess of 60 days.

The average number of days credit taken by clients can be calculated from balance sheet debtors x 365 divided by turnover.

Look at the Trends

The first stage in preparing the financial side of a practice business plan is to examine the available financial and management accounts and to record trends for the following parameters during the last three available financial years.

REVENUE. Practice revenue in real terms (taking into account the impact of inflation over the period).

PROFITS. Owner's profit as a percentage of revenue, as a return on investment and in financial terms (do not forget the impact of inflation).

COSTS. Major cost headings as a percentage of revenue.

RATIOS

- liquidity (working capital and acid test)
- stock turnover (times per annum)
- debtor turnover (days)
- gearing

Now write down a summary of your perception of the practice's financial strengths and weaknesses as a result of the exercise.

Planning for Profit

Now that you have prepared a brief but comprehensive financial report based on historical information, the much more exciting and stimulating exercise follows. You must decide where you want the business to get to in financial terms over the next two years. This is not the time to be vague. A general promise to yourself to seek to improve profits or to generate additional turnover is not good enough and frankly is unlikely to happen. You will have to be much more positive and specific. You may decide for example to increase the profit level by 50% in real terms over the next two years or to improve stock turnover levels from 8 to 12 times per annum over the next twelve months. Consider all the possible objectives for your practice.

The approach of many veterinary practice owners to profit is a strange one. For many the question has nothing to do with profit as a financial measure of performance but a subjective judgment. 'As long as I can draw the cash I need to maintain my personal and family needs I'm really not too bothered about the accounts'. Perhaps that is why there seems to be little urgency in providing the practice accountant with the data required to prepare the accounts. In turn accountants are under little pressure to prepare a draft set. As a result, the practice accountant eventually produces a draft set of accounts some months after the financial year end. Practice owners then check turnover to see how much it has increased over the previous year. They note their costs and accept the bottom line figure — the profit — with pleasure, mild interest or horror.

If you are a veterinary practice owner who has decided to prepare a comprehensive business plan which includes specific financial targets, you will surely take a different approach.

The Budget

i) Decide AT THE OUTSET how much profit you need to make next year.
ii) What do you know about your level of practice costs? You can forecast quite accurately what your fixed costs are likely to be next year and the year after and you know how your variable costs will be related to the number of cases seen next year.
iii) Now calculate the level of turnover which the practice will need to generate to achieve the predetermined level of profit.

Now you will be embarking on a budget making process. Not a task which incorporates some vague hopes about practice turnover but a detailed identifiable strategy to ensure that the turnover is achieved. Easier said than done maybe, but let us have a closer look at the reality.

Profit is the difference between the value of the work carried out during a specific period of time and the costs involved in doing so. It follows that the only way to increase profits is to reduce the costs or increase the value of the services rendered.

The Theory

Look more closely at the options and consider the difference between costs which are 'fixed', i.e.

which are likely to remain about the same if the volume of work increases or decreases within a limited band of say 25% and those costs which are variable, i.e. are related directly to the number of cases seen.

The major cost items in most practices are the cost of drugs and professional supplies and the cost of salaries and wages. Assume that all other costs are fixed by volume or incurred by necessity. Consider a hypothetical practice generating 100 units of turnover, with fixed costs at 50 units and variable costs at 20% of revenue. The practice generates a profit of 30 units. The picture can be summarised as follows:

Turnover	100
Less Costs	
Fixed costs	50
Variable costs (20%)	20

Total costs	70

Profit	30

What Determines the Profit?

CONSIDER:
i) What measures can we take to improve turnover?

The total practice income is simply the total number of transactions during a period of time (the case volume) multiplied by the average value of each of those transactions (average transaction value). So we can:

- increase fees or prices
- increase case volume
- increase the services rendered or goods supplied per transaction.

ii) What measures can we take to affect fixed costs?

Monitor fixed costs at least monthly. Eliminate waste and then make sure that the fixed costs really are fixed over the specific period of time.
iii) What measures can we take to affect variable costs?

Monitor variable costs at least monthly and ensure that they remain within budgeted limits per transaction.

iv) What then would be the impact on profits? if for example we;

- increased case volume by 5%?
- increased the services rendered per transaction by 5%?
- and increased the fees by 5%?

and at the same time we took steps to ensure that fixed costs remain fixed and that variable costs remain at 20% of revenue.

Here is the sum:

Turnover	115
Less Costs	
Fixed costs	50
Variable costs (20%)	23

Total costs	73

Profit	42

which represents an increased profit level of 40%

FUN ISN'T IT!

The Reality

Some may say that's all very well in theory. It certainly would not work in my practice. Why not? Let's have a look at a hypothetical single-handed practice with a turnover of say £135,000 generating £40,000 for the owner. He decides to increase his profit to £60,000 within two years. What steps could he take to achieve that target?

Suppose that in the first year he decides to increase fees by 5%, plans to increase case volume by 2.5% and increases the value of the average transaction by only 2.5% (remember these increases are net of value added or other sales taxes and ignore the impact of inflation). He further decides to maintain the fixed costs at £65,300 and to reduce the variable costs to 20% of revenue. Assuming that he achieves those targets (surely not unreasonable), what would be the outcome?

Here are the figures:

	THIS YEAR £	NEXT YEAR £
Turnover	135,000	148,500
Less Costs		
Fixed costs	65,300	65,300
Variable costs	(22%) 29,700	(20%) 29,700
Total costs	95,000	95,000
	------	------
Profit	40,000	53,500

representing an increase of 33% by the end of year 1. Well on target!

FUN ISN'T IT?

What do you need to know about your own practice to do similar sums?

Not too much and your accountant will certainly be able to help you. You will need to identify your:

- fixed costs
- variable costs and
- case volume

We cannot over-emphasise the crucial importance of monitoring case volume and thus the value of your average transaction.

The detailed budgeting procedure is a lot more complicated than suggested. But for now, take some paper and a pen and explore some figures for your own practice. Just see what you can achieve as a result of relatively small changes in fees, case volume, average transaction values, fixed and variable costs. Perhaps you will get as enthusiastic about the process as we are!

Your Budget

Here are some general comments which may help when you start to put together your financial plan — the budget for your practice.

Plan for profit. Profits don't just happen they are made. The amount of profit a practice makes will depend on the quality of the decisions made and the control measures used to work to the plan. That plan is usually called the budget. Be wise not to regard the budget so much as what will happen come what may, but as a statement of what is intended to happen.

Budgeting provides the practitioner with a detailed step by step (monthly or quarterly) route to the target set for the practice. Budgeting is as important for the smallest practice as it is for large enterprises.

At this stage the budget is for dreamers. Play with it. Consider 'what would happen if' and do the sums to find out. When complete, your budget will incorporate a number of target figures which should be realistic, but not necessarily easily attainable.

Planning

Use the data collected to plan for the future. Consider budgeting. Involve everybody in the practice. Assign responsibilities to named individuals to analyse the changes that have occurred in their own department and come up with proposals for improvement. Ask them to identify what they can achieve over the next two years and what resources they will require to achieve them. Ask them to come up with free thinking, creative, and productive alternatives to the present way things are done in their department. Ensure that their proposals are well thought out, written down, costed and include a timetable and targets.

Much of the budget will be concerned with practice revenue and about using staff resources to generate additional income. It would not be realistic for an owner simply to set targets and then to instruct the staff to achieve them. It has to be a team effort in which the owner takes the lead. At a fairly early stage, involve the whole team in discussing fee levels, cost control, revenue generation and in setting targets. After that, the owners/managers leadership qualities will be required to motivate colleagues to achieve and to beat the projections.

There are a couple of ways of dealing with inflation when preparing a budget. Either ignore it and show all figures at current prices or make some judgment about expected inflation rates and apply them in the calculations. Include a note in the budget to indicate what assumptions have been made and remember to include a figure for contingencies — not too small and not too large.

Other Financial Tools

Break Even Analysis

Preparation of a break-even analysis chart is a convenient way of examining all those factors which will effect practice profitability. Figure 3 illustrates the various components:

- case/transaction volume
- fixed costs
- variable costs
- revenue.

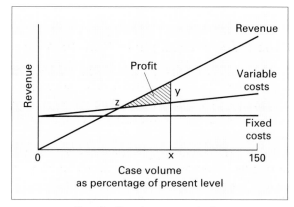

FIG. 3   Break-even analysis.

The points:
x = case volume at which the practice is operating
y = profit level
z = break-even point

Break-even analysis can be used to examine practice sensitivity to changes in case volume and changes in fees as the following examples illustrate. (The figures are derived from the projected figures for the practice referred to on page 81).

> turnover   £148,500
> fixed costs   £65,300
> variable costs   £29,700
> case volume   10,607
> average transaction value   £14.00
> variable cost per unit   £2.80

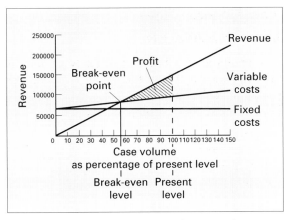

FIG. 4   Sensitivity to change in case volume.

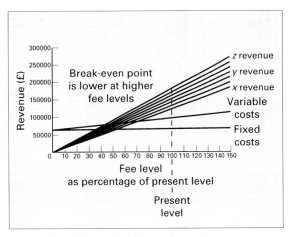

FIG. 5   Sensitivity to change in fees.

Sensitivity to Changes in Case Volume

Figure 4 illustrates a break even analysis to demonstrate the sensitivity of the projections to changes in transaction volume ranging from say 70% to 130% of the projected volume of 10,607.

Break even data suggest that if case volume during the projected twelve months were to vary while all other factors were to remain unchanged, the impact on practice profitability would be as follows:

Case Volume	Practice profit
70%	17,860 (approx)
80%	29,740 (approx)
90%	41,620 (approx)
100%	53,500 (approx)
110%	65,380 (approx)
120%	77,260 (approx)
130%	89,140 (approx)

Sensitivity to Changes in Fees

A second break even analysis (Figure 5) demonstrates the sensitivity of the projections to changes in practice fees ranging from 70% to 130% of the existing fees as follows:

Assume that management accounting information indicates that overall practice income is derived as follows: 65% from professional fees and 35% from the sale/dispensing of medication. On this basis the following data has been incorporated in the analysis: (note; ATV = average transaction value).

Revenue slopes on the attached graphics represent:
Slope X Fees at 70% of existing level
Slope Y Fees at 100% of existing level
Slope Z Fees at 130% of existing level
Break even analysis data suggest that if practice fees during the projected twelve months were to vary while all other factors were to remain

% of existing fee	fee £	drugs £	ATV	Vol	revenue £
70	6.37	4.90	11.27	10,607	119,540
80	7.28	4.90	12.18	10,607	129,193
90	8.19	4.90	13.09	10,607	138,845
100	9.10	4.90	14.00	10,607	148,500
110	10.01	4.90	14.91	10,607	158,150
120	10.92	4.90	15.82	10,607	167,802
130	11.83	4.90	16.73	10,607	177,455

unchanged, the impact on practice profitability would be as follows:

Profit
Fees at 70% of existing level £24,540 (approx)
Fees at 100% of existing level £53,500 (approx)
Fees at 130% of existing level £82,455 (approx)

In reality, marked fee changes may have an effect on case volume. It is a management task to judge the significance of the likely impact. The level and direction of demand, i.e., case volume changes, depends to some extent on the market segment being served. While significant fee increases may marginally depress volume in the cost conscious end of the market, they may result in an additional demand in the segment where clients equate quality with price.

Remember:

i) the steeper the slope the more rapid the change in profits in response to case volume and,

ii) you can also quickly demonstrate the impact in profits on changes in your fixed costs. Why not try it? Consider for example the impact on the profits above if the practice were to employ an additional receptionist at say £8,000 (an increase of fixed costs by £8,000) and a decline of case volume by say 10%.

A Few Rules

A few simple rules about BUDGETING are worth remembering:

- Spend as much time as you need to prepare and refine your practice budget. Having done so use it. Refer to it regularly. Don't file it away and forget it.
- It is far easier to budget for expenditure than for revenue. But, it is much more fun and creative to budget for revenue than costs.
- Effective budgeting depends on regular monitoring of practice performance. Management steps must be taken to correct adverse trends and adjust the plan as necessary.
- Take action when you identify a problem.
- You can't plan for the totally unexpected. Most problems, however, seem to arise

in practices which lack any sort of plan. However formal or informal, the plan establishes where a practice is going and how it is going to get there.

- Finally, there are only four ways in which to increase practice profits:

i) reduce the fixed or variable costs.

ii) raise the revenue per transaction by increasing fees or by providing additional services or goods.

iii) increase the volume of transactions

iv) or a combination of any of these.

Controlling Costs

Reducing costs logically comes first because, or so it is said, money saved is better than money earned.

Reduce Waste

Cost reduction implies the identification and elimination of waste. This includes waste of money, stock, time or any other scarce resources. There must be a constant search for ways of improving productivity.

Try and approach the problem in a logical way and write your ideas down as you go along. Start now to prepare a list of ways in which resources are wasted in your practice:

What materials do you and your staff waste? Think of all the possibilities such as medicines, dressings, cleaning material, cotton wool, disinfectant, X-Ray film, paper and record cards. What about time? Are your staff members adding to the practice overhead costs or do they see themselves as actively, directly or indirectly, generating additional revenue to produce more profit in which they will share?

Take your practice manager, head nurse or senior receptionist into your confidence. Ask them to prepare a list of ways in which they think money or resources are wasted in the practice. Make it clear that you do not want them to name individual names but you might well offer some incentive for the best suggestion within say the next week, for reducing waste in the practice and measuring the improvement.

Managing Cash Flow and Credit

Early on in life we were all taught that saving some of our money was the way to grow wealthy. As we became more sophisticated in financial matters we discovered that leverage was the tool for financial gain. It seemed easy. The secret was to use 'other peoples money' to purchase assets which then appreciated in value. Recession over the past three years has reminded us of the truth of what we were taught in childhood and practices that have adopted a conservative attitude towards debt were those that could survive recession most easily.

The lesson we learned so well when we were young is the importance of cash in hand. The lesson we have to keep reminding ourselves about now is the importance of planning for and monitoring cash flow and of management control.

Consider an example in which a branch practice was managed by an employee veterinarian. He had complete management discretion for the satellite unit including purchasing, paying all creditors, hiring and firing and so on. Everything seemed fine. The practice owner monitored the bank balance, receipts and payments. After a few months however, he started to receive complaints from creditors. Their bills were not being paid. He discovered to his horror that the practice had built up a very high level of debtors and stock and that there was a pile of unpaid bills.

What was the problem? The main problem was a lack of control. Practice growth had been satisfactory but the owner had not bothered to monitor debtors, stock levels or incurred expenses.

What were the lessons he learned?

- Whatever management structure is in operation, it is important for the practice owner to establish an effective management accounting control system to ensure that all the information he needs is available as and when he wants it.
- Include in your regular management information system turnover, case volume, receipts, debtors (including aged debtors), creditors (including aged creditors) and actual stock levels.

- Practice liquidity is most important and many accountants would advise typical small animal practices to hold a sum in their current account equivalent to at least 1% to 1.5% of gross income in cash.
- Remember too the importance of planning for overdraft or other credit facilities well in advance of your likely need.
- Manage your payments and monitor your current bank balance. Some practice owners are pastmasters at timing their payments. Those vendors that offer discounts are paid immediately while others, that work on net 30 day payments, are deferred. Good hearted vendors will excuse momentary cash problems and offer free credit but their good nature should not be abused. Remember how you feel when a client delays payment to you.
- Intelligent stock management can help to ease your cash flow problems. Examine your purchasing policies. Do you have too many product lines on the shelf or is it time to rationalise them? Be aware of the danger of building up a stock of outdated products which will never be used. Consider a policy of only taking on a new product at the cost of dropping another.
- Establish a minimum stock holding for each product but review it regularly. Remember that the staff member responsible for stock ordering will tend to err on the side of ordering too much rather than not enough.

Profit and cashflow are terms which are often misunderstood. Cashflow relates to the amount of profit that is available to be distributed. The balance of the profit is used to purchase stock, to lend to debtors, purchase equipment or pay off debt. All of these transactions divert precious profit away from the practice owner and into the hands of the bank, clients or vendors. Cash is one of the most valuable of assets. Other assets are also important but creditors like to see a practice with enough liquid cash so that they feel confident that they will be paid. The recession has taught many creditors that the balance sheet with a strong asset position is meaningless unless enough assets can be readily converted to cash.

More businesses go bankrupt because they run out of cash than those which fail because they can't make a profit. Veterinary practices are cash hungry and rapidly expanding practices are most susceptible to a chronic lack of cash. In some cases growing practices have tried to support a debtors figure (receivables) of up to ten or twenty percent of the total fee income for the year. Unless the owner has sufficient personal wealth to loan back to the practice, bankruptcy is just around the corner. This occurs when veterinarians cannot honour obligations because so much of their cash is tied up in debtors. Have a searching look at how much it costs to lend client's money for a week or a month or more free, when you are running an overdraft on your current account.

Too often practices with a high debtor level (receivables) rationalise that once the major debtors start to settle their accounts they will be wealthy. The hope can persist for months. All too often the bulk of long term receivables become bad debts and have to be written off.

One of the major reasons why the debtor situation goes awry is because the practices have an inadequate credit control system in operation. An effective control system must incorporate a number of principles. Firstly receivables have to be controlled before the service is provided. The problem is not an easy one in veterinary practice but every client who runs an account must be aware that, once the credit limit is reached, no further service will be provided by your practice until payment is received. Secondly, veterinarians must take a more realistic view of the need for growth. It is great to increase average transaction values and case volume but not if each case makes an inadequate contribution to profits and a negative contribution to cash flow. It is not the number of clients that is meaningful for the practice but the quality of those clients as contributors to the bottom line. If you are not paid for the services you provide for some clients, you may find yourself in a situation where you are unable to provide any services for any clients. Thirdly, the practice owner must keep a 'hands on' approach to credit control. They must be intimately involved in the practice on a day to day basis. Stewardship of a veterinary practice from a distance may be regarded as a being design for failure.

Purchasing Policy

What about your own purchasing policies? How do you react to special offers, discounts or goods in lieu? Are you tempted or do you calculate the impact on your own profit or cash flow. Remember that the profitability of your stock keeping function depends on the percentage margin and the frequency with which stock is rotated.

Charging for Your Services

Many veterinarians feel guilty about charging and may even apologise for the fee as they hand over an invoice. If you are sure that the procedure recommended was necessary, that the job was carried out properly, that every aspect of the case was discussed with the client, do not feel guilty! Fees are based on your professional knowledge, skill and experience and take into account all the costs of providing quality services. Self confidence about personal abilities and those of your staff demand that you charge an appropriate fee. If anything needs to be said it is that 'I'm pleased to says that we can offer this standard of service for ....

Prepare a detailed fee schedule, date it and review it at least quarterly. Every member of the staff must understand the fee schedule and under what circumstances service fees should be charged. Most veterinary practices offer occasional services to children or the very old, or treat wild birds and mammals at little or no cost. These exceptions must be an established part of the overall policy. Establish a business-like procedure to eliminate errors and the tendency of the consulting veterinarian to reduce or waive the fees other than in these accepted circumstances.

One of the advantages of computer based systems is that the total fee for a particular client is calculated automatically from a predetermined fee schedule. Always render an invoice at the time of service. If using a manual system use multi-copied, sequentially numbered, invoices for control purposes. Worksheets which aren't completed and priced until later in the day, or indeed some days later, will nearly always underestimate the value of the services rendered and stock items dispensed.

Cash, cheque and credit card receipts must be reconciled with the day-book, till printout or computer summary at least daily. Remember that no matter how good a fee and invoicing system is, it will be valueless if the data is not converted into cash.

A practice strategy for fee setting is an important component of the practice budget making process. Determine a positive policy for fees. Establish a rationale for determining fees for new services. Lastly, develop a routine as part of the management accounting system in the practice to monitor the adequacy of your prices.

There are a number of approaches to fee setting:

i) A mathematical approach which is based on cost accounting methods and which involves identifying the required total fee income, calculating the available work chargeable hours during a period and thus determining an hourly charge. The charge per service is then based on the time involved in providing it.

ii) system which is based merely on what the competition is doing. Some practices maintain their fees at the average of the other practices in the area or they decide positively to be a little above or a little below their competitors. The problem here is that such a policy is merely reactive and if the majority of practices in the area are cautious and nervous as far as fees are concerned it will result in veterinary fee levels in the area declining further and further below realistic levels.

iii) A third approach is based on the view that fee setting is an art form in which consideration is given to how strongly the client needs and values what you are selling, how much he can afford to pay, what alternative choices he or she may have and the extent to which the client is prepared to shop around. At the same time the veterinarian needs to know what sum is required to cover the fixed and variable costs in providing the service and what contribution that service is required to make towards practice profits.

The owners of the practice must decide at the outset the objective of the enterprise. If you are determined to control your practice, decide the financial and time commitment you are prepared to invest, then determine the profit required. You will now appreciate that fee levels should be designed to maximise profit rather than turnover.

There is an old saying that when 5% of clients threaten to take their business away because prices are too high and when 2% do, fees are about right. If nobody complains vigorously that fees are too high, be quite sure that they are too low. If increasing fees to a level at which 5% do take their business away, the message should not be to reduce charges but to take steps to increase the perceived value of the service provided.

Fee setting is a matter of considerable interest to veterinarians in practice. Consider the following thoughts:

No single practice can satisfy all the people all the time. Trying to do so may end up by no one being satisfied. Consumers in the 1990s will be more demanding and have more choice than ever before. Clients who in the past have been satisfied with reasonable levels of service at reasonable fees will be in the minority. Many will decide to go 'up market', i.e., they will search for the very highest standards of care and quality and will be prepared to pay the price. Others will become increasingly cost conscious. Clients will be more concerned with value for money but will still demand a quality service.

Here are some more questions:

- Are you enjoying the job that you are doing?
- Is the practice generating sufficient revenue so that you can pay your staff well and give them sufficient leisure time to maintain their enthusiasm for the job?
- Is the practice achieving a sufficient level of profit to plough back into the business?
- Are you satisfied with your 'take home pay'?

If you have doubts about any of the answers there may well be a case for a significant increase in your fees as long as that policy is matched by a real improvement in the perceived value of the services you provide. Do not be defensive. Be positive and be sure that you and your staff are proud of your prices and that your practice image is one of value for money. It really doesn't matter whether your fee for a particular service is £10, $50 or ECU100 as long as the perceived value is £11, $55 or ECU120.

It is probably true that veterinary practice owners are paid exactly what they think they are worth. Only when veterinarians are totally convinced that the services they provide are worth a great deal more will their clients begin to agree. A management consultant to the veterinary profession recently said that he had never ever come across a practice where raising fees had not increased net income and that he had yet to see any significant decline in volume either. Price is an important element in a clients decision to buy. But, perceived care, interest and quality are much more important to those clients you want to keep.

Data Input and Retrieval

Effective financial management depends entirely on the accuracy and completeness of the financial and other information which is available. It is essential therefore to select and establish an appropriate data input and retrieval system which will satisfy the particular requirements of the practice.

It wasn't so many years ago that bookkeeping entries in veterinary practice were maintained entirely in ledgers or on ledger sheets stored in cumbersome, heavily-bound volumes. More recently, veterinary practices have upgraded their approach to the accumulation of information. A variety of 'one- write' manual systems to allocate costs to a number of specific cost headings and to identify sources of revenue have been developed and used successfully in veterinary practice. Some of these have been used in conjunction with the batch input of data through computer service bureaux to provide monthly and annual financial information.

Cash receipts followed the same pattern. They were recorded using the same type of 'one-write' system. Some progressive practices utilised 'one write' invoice systems in which carbon strips

on NCR paper were used to record entries simultaneously on ledger sheets beneath. At the same time, electronic accounting tools have evolved from electronic cash registers to 'in-house' micro-computers powered by sophisticated operating systems and user-friendly menus for data accumulation and retrieval. Although some practices still use batch entry processing systems, on line computer processing is much more common in those practices which have invested in computer technology.

Selecting an Accounting System

Practice owners and managers need to consider a wide range of factors in defining the needs of the practice for data recording and retrieval systems. They include the technology available, the management need for internal control, the level of accuracy required and the likely capital and revenue costs. Also involved is the enthusiasm and competence of the individuals who will be required to operate the system. Mechanised systems provide much greater internal control but their cost and level of sophistication is also greater. Security is also a factor and there may be advantages in separating the responsibility of individuals providing the service from those who record the transaction. Electronic systems can do this and also provide a range of other safeguards such as passwords, multiple screen options and a range of possible access levels.

However, internal control systems cost money. Mechanised systems provide a greater degree of security, but also demand an initial investment that may be far more costly than some veterinarians are willing to spend. For example, a stand alone computer system that might cost somewhere around $5,000, can be used to maintain a record of debtors (receivables), generate a summary of payments made and maintain and monitor a number of management ratios and indices. A spreadsheet might be considered an extravagant expenditure by a veterinarian establishing a new practice. On the other hand, a simple 'one write' manual accounting and recording system with a card index for client and patient records purchased for a few hundred dollars (capable of maintaining receipts and payments) may be far more costly in the long term as a result of the system's lack of inherent internal control. The cost of periodic supplies for the manual system may be far less than the maintenance costs for a computer system's software and hardware, computer supplies and personnel training. On the other hand, the possible income lost because of inadequate clinical reminder systems, failure to charge properly for all the services rendered or from fraud, may far exceed the cost of maintaining a more sophisticated electronic system.

Provided the practice owner has prepared a detailed specification of practice requirements and the computer vendor has anticipated the needs of the veterinary client, a computer system can provide a far better system of internal control. It is more accurate. It can summarise financial and other data in multiple categories with greater ease and lower long-term costs. In the long run, it is more cost effective because it decreases the amount of time needed by the practice accountant to summarise accounting information and it provides the practice manager with the information required for intelligent, informative, and timely decisions.

Once a computer based accounting and recording system is established, the time taken by support staff members in administrative chores will be reduced. As a result, staff time will be used more efficiently and, given good management, will be much more productive. Do not assume that improved efficiency will result in a reduction in pay-roll costs. You will find that pay-roll will increase rather than decrease but the information available for management will be far more sophisticated and useful than before. The responsibility of management is to understand how to utilise that investment and increase efficiency in generating significant increases in profits. Much of that increase will be derived from the opportunities for increased client contact and internal marketing opportunities and from maintaining a much closer control of practice costs.

The Benefits of a Computer

Timeliness of information is a critical factor in determining an appropriate accounting/recording system for veterinary practice. News becomes aged and decays with time. Financial information must be recent and accurate to be valuable. With 'one-write' systems, cheque details for example, are recorded on a general summary sheet as they are written. It is then necessary to prepare summary purchase ledger information before it can be of value for management accounting purposes. This activity is very labour intensive.

A computer system on the other hand utilises the efficiency of data entry to minimise employee involvement in preparing summary information. As invoice details are keyed in to a purchase ledger programme, the creditor is automatically established in a queue for payment and the information can be posted automatically to a general and nominal ledger programme. All of these steps are done automatically with very little operator input and result in a high level of accuracy and reliability.

Computerisation provides for the manipulation of data, which only has to be keyed into the system once, to provide management accounting information in a form and at a frequency required by management. The cost for that convenience is paid in advance through the acquisition of the capital asset and software. Paper and pen systems on the other hand, can be set up quickly and cheaply but become costly because of the continuous stationery supplies needed, the labour required to maintain them and their predisposition to error and even fraud.

Many practice owners can remember the hours that were spent every day attempting to reconcile a cash receipts journal on paper or 'one write' system. Sometimes the amount of cash in the cash drawer or till did not match the summary of cash that was shown from the day book receipts. All too often mathematical errors, transposed numbers, slipped decimal points, or general lack of care and diligence resulted in inaccuracies which were difficult and extremely time consuming to resolve.

Electronic systems overcome many of these problems. With most veterinary practice software systems, cash reconciliation is instantaneous and automatic. Mathematical errors are eliminated and cash receipts, by various modes of payment (cash, bank card, cheque or credit card) are recorded instantaneously. This level of efficiency and the improved productivity of support staff time may alone justify the cost of the capital acquisition of the equipment.

Don't be fooled. The initial cost for the installation is only the start. Bear in mind the ongoing costs of complying with the system needs. Hardware systems require service agreements. Software systems require either update payments or software service contracts. Every change in software also demands new learning skills by the operators. A computer system with multiple updates is more costly to maintain than a computer system with few updates. Undoubtedly the system worth having is worth maintaining, but it is necessary to assess the maintenance and service contract costs by comparing the benefits of purchasing one system rather than another.

It is our view that, except in the smallest of practices, manual accounting and recording systems are not even a logical choice in today's computerised society. The question of maintaining clinical records is perhaps a different issue and many veterinary practice owners have successfully installed computerised accounting and recording systems which they use in conjunction with manual, handwritten clinical records on a traditional card record system. Once they are convinced of the value, the effectiveness and efficiency of the electronic system, transfer of clinical records to the computer is the logical next step. A computer based system and clinical record cards will be used side by side for the first few months but it is surprising how quickly the card system becomes almost completely redundant.

The highest importance should be placed on the 'user friendly' attributes of software programmes. Consider the degree of training required for operators when purchasing very sophisticated programs. Frequently, the individual who buys the computer system is not ultimately responsible for using it regularly and making it work successfully. The person who makes the purchase decision may be attracted by the options, features and management report capabilities while forgetting that the operators who will use the system may be incapable of handling the sophisticated features.

Choosing a System

The best approach to the possible purchase of a computer based accounting and recording system for your practice is;

i) Take your practice to pieces! Go through your existing manual system in some detail. Consider every piece of paper, every form and every book and ledger which you and your staff complete painstakingly. Review what is required. Precisely what information will you, your colleagues, your staff, your accountant, your bank manager, government agencies and others need? When will you and they need it? Why? What will be done with it? What management, clerical, clinical, marketing or other decisions could you, should you or might you take as a result?

ii) Draw up a detailed specification of your management, accounting and recording system for the future. Forget the most appropriate tools at this stage. Simply concentrate on the information which is or might be available. How, why and when you need it and what will you do with it when you have it?

iii) Now consider the most appropriate tools required to carry out the task. Pen and ink, paper, record cards, typewriters, calculators, word processors, spreadsheets, databases and computer hardware, printers, copiers and so on. You will then appreciate that a computer is simply a tool. An expensive and demanding tool, but nonetheless a tool which may, or may not, assist you to manage your practice more effectively, economically and efficiently.

iv) Now is the time to draw up a detailed specification for your practice for computer software, hardware and peripherals. Despatch it with a covering letter to a number of suppliers. Ask them to identify how closely their products will match your specification, at what capital costs and at what ongoing maintenance costs including training.

In some instances, practice managers attempt to force the practice to conform to a particular computer system. This approach may sometimes be appropriate. There is always human resistance to change but if the practice personnel are not competent to handle the new system or if their level of resistance is too great, the computer system will be doomed to failure from the outset. Sometimes the biggest impediment to the successful introduction of a computer based system in veterinary practice is the practice principal or owner. This is particularly true if the individual feels coerced by peer or sales pressure to make the investment, but does not trust the system and has no intention of complying with the discipline required or of trying to understand its attributes. They may be secretly delighted if sooner or later the system is regarded as a failure so that they can say 'I told you so'.

The Importance of Security

When choosing any accounting system, consider the available security options. With manual, handwritten systems, security is at its lowest level. The highest probability of misappropriation will occur when internal controls are the weakest. Fraud is much more difficult and much less likely with a properly designed computer software system complete with the appropriate internal management controls.

It will be necessary to determine the 'need-to-know' levels for all employees for access to the system. Providing all members of a practice with computerised password override options may facilitate multiple access to data for quick response to client needs. That same facility could become a problem if an unscrupulous individual were to use the information to manipulate data to disguise fraud. As veterinary practices become bigger, busier and more successful, you will sooner or later come across a dishonest employee. You should certainly bear the possibility in mind when you are contemplating major capital investment in a computer based management accounting system.

Security extends well beyond the idea of theft of data or cash. Computer systems can occasionally crash with the possible loss of all your valuable data. Computerisation provides the opportunity to back up data electronically for safe storage elsewhere. Manual systems are not, in the normal course of operations, photocopied and stored off-site and a properly managed computer system can provide a greater level of protection in the event of disaster.

Financial Information

Financial information is only of value for management purposes if it is relevant, accurate, reliable and consistent. This ensures that comparison with previous periods is valid. Similar attributes are necessary to compare business performance with other businesses in the same market sector. Interpractice comparison, subject to anonymity and confidentiality for specific individuals or enterprises, can be of considerable benefit for veterinary practice. Like must be compared with like and great steps have been taken by the American Animal Hospital Association and others over the last few years. The AAHA has published a codified chart of accounts to standardise financial accounting information for veterinary practices on a world-wide basis. The chart of accounts was designed to accommodate manual and computerised systems and to maintain the integrity of data, for example for specific statutory requirements, between countries. Financial statements, management reports and tax summaries can be prepared dependent on the requirements of that specific country's generally accepted accounting principles and governmental regulations. Nominal code classifications can be re-numbered providing the basic classification captions maintain their integrity. Sufficient latitude has been established within the numbering system of the Chart of Accounts to accommodate more detailed analysis.

The choice of an appropriate accounting system must also be sensitive to the type of practice that will use it. A small animal practice, for example, may have uniquely different system requirements than an equine practice. Mixed practices will also have particular requirements. Referral practices in specific disciplines like orthopaedics, dermatology, ophthalmology, internal medicine and oncology will probably not depend so much on an effective reminder system within the software programme as on the ability to monitor and maintain contact with colleagues on referral issues.

General Ledger

In the general ledger portion of the system, the selection of the appropriate account headings will depend upon the methodology for income and expense recognition. A cash basis of accounting will clearly demand a far simpler system than an accrual basis. A cash basis of accounting is one which recognises items of income and expenditure only when payment is received or paid. An accrual basis of accounting generally recognises income when it is earned but not necessarily received, and expenses when they are incurred but not necessarily paid.

Capturing financial data is costly. You really only need to record and retrieve non clinical information which is required either by your advisers and other third parties or for management purposes. Accumulating detailed categories of income and expenditure that are seldom if ever used, is an expensive waste. Your aim should be to utilise the fewest number of man hours to acquire the information needed as accurately as possible.

Select a manual or computer based system that meets the unique needs of your practice. Consider the capital and revenue costs and its 'user friendly' attributes. Will it record and retrieve what you want? Consider whether its level of sophistication will match your needs and abilities and those of your staff. Will it be accurate, timely and reliable?

Data accumulation costs money. Acquire the best usable information and consider the possible need to compromise about unnecessary detail. Ensure that the selection of an appropriate system in not in the hands of one individual, particularly if that individual is you! Seek plenty of advice. Prepare a specification for a system that will meet your needs and work through a detailed selection process along the lines we have suggested. The opportunity costs lost in selecting the wrong system will far outweigh your initial investment.

Computer Generated Reports

The detailed specification which should be prepared before finally deciding which veterinary software package to purchase should include your needs for reports for management purposes.

Consider the following as a guide;

- Stock control, stock usage and stockholding.
- Client invoicing with day end summary and revenue analysis by service, product, patient species or veterinarian.
- Payment receipts with end of day summary.
- Audit trails to trace errors.
- Control of missed charges.
- Improved patient records.
- Legible records.
- Improved communication.

Period End and Annual Reports for Management

- Cost headings as a percentage of turnover.
- Veterinarian and support staff productivity.
- Monitor number of new clients and clients lost.
- Client origin (referral, yellow pages).
- Aged debtors and creditors.
- Case volume.
- Average transaction value.
- Data trends and comparison with same month last year.

General Ledger Programme

A general ledger programme designed to identify cost headings under a number of categories will enable the practice manager and others to monitor cost heading trends in financial terms and as a percentage of gross, to recognise adverse trends at an early stage and to take appropriate corrective action.

The programme will record each item of expenditure with date, invoice and cheque number and nominal ledger classification. It can be used as a reminder system for insurance and subscription renewals, bank standing orders and direct debit information.

Internal Control

As practices become larger and busier and as staff numbers increase it will be increasingly important to consider security measures to reduce the unpleasant but realistic possibility of internal dishonesty.

Internal Controls are the safety features established within an accounting system to safeguard practice assets and to mitigate liabilities.

Safeguard Your Assets

Cash and Receivables

The practice balance sheet identifies those assets that can be subject to internal control. Cash and cash equivalents can be controlled in a variety of ways, mainly through separating staff duties so that the person who has control of the asset does not have control of the records. For example, the person who opens the mail would not be the same person who records receipts.

The accounts receivable system should be examined for extraordinary adjustments. Banking should be done daily and a separate person should control and reconcile cash receipts with the day book. Computer generated reports should always agree with the daily cash receipts count and a specific individual should be responsible for ensuring that they do. Do not ignore or accept differences, even minor ones. Develop a reputation in the practice for being a stickler for accuracy and ensure that errors are identified and corrected by the individual staff member responsible for them. Be tough but be fair.

On an annual basis, the opening accounts receivable (debtors) balance, the fees earned throughout the year and total cash receipts, should be reconciled by the practice manager and signed off before forwarding the books to the practice accountant.

Cash is critical. The practice manager should insist on an impressed petty cash account (a system in which petty cash is only replenished to the extent of receipts received for reimbursement). A single individual should be responsible for maintaining and monitoring petty cash and any errors or discrepancies should be reported and resolved promptly.

Review your payroll figures on a regular basis to compare costs as a percentage of your gross income. Staff who think that they are paid inadequately may complain, may leave or may start to steal from the practice because they are able to rationalise some degree of justification for their dishonesty. Keep your honest employees honest by establishing and monitoring an effective cash control system.

Be aware of other possible methods which have been used by employees to steal cash. They include manipulating client accounts in a variety of ways to indicate that account balances have been paid while the cash finds its way into employee pockets, cheques identified on the purchase ledger but with an incorrect payee name, forging a signature and banking the cheque and relying on inadequate control systems to take small sums from the cash drawer or from petty cash.

Since 44% of all employee thefts occur at the cash register, attention to cash receipts is critical. Insist that all clients are given a receipt. Clients thus become part of your defence against employees not ringing up a correct transaction. Pre-numbered or computer generated receipts are also extremely useful in maintaining internal control.

REMEMBER — theft can occur from other than cash.

Stock and Supplies

Theft of stock and supplies by staff or clients can occur in a number of ways.

Consider a few.

An employee purchases a case of dog food when the reception area is quiet. They ring up the transaction but they record an amount that is considerably less than the actual price. The difference remains in the employees pocket. That is theft.

Clients or staff members come into the reception or stock area on some pretext and simply take items of stock. Such theft can be very difficult to spot but much can be learned by monitoring stock order lists and keeping a close and perhaps random watch on invoices to spot any unusual ordering pattern.

Keep a particularly close watch on dietary products and analyse them separately on your chart of accounts. Dog and cat foods are favourite products for theft from veterinary practice.

Controlled drugs are critical to the proper management of veterinary hospitals and their storage and use demand specific security and control measures. Be sure that your practice complies with every statutory requirement for controlled substances. Theft of controlled drugs by criminal factions outside the practice is always a possibility but employees too can be a possible risk. There have been instances of employees who are under such emotional stress that they use controlled drugs from a veterinary pharmacy to commit suicide.

What about office supplies? Be reasonable. If an employee needs an extra pen, he may carelessly slip it in his pocket and go home. A degree of 'slippage' is acceptable. On the other hand wholesale loss of items such as reams of paper, boxes of pens or pencils, packets of paper clips, numbers of books and packs of stationery and unauthorised personal use of the telephone or fax, is most certainly not acceptable and must be stopped.

Your Clients and Your Time

What other of your practice assets may be stolen? What about the theft of your clients by employees? Groomers and professional staff have been known to use client lists belonging to their employers to attract customers for their own commercial use. Receptionists have been known to steal by securing employment in another practice and giving client lists away to the new employer. Photocopying client and patient records, and accessing computers to copy data files are all examples of theft. You should be aware of the possibility, however unlikely, in your own practice.

Inefficient staff, or staff who are simply idle, steal time from their employers. In busy small animal practices with a number of staff members, employees can simply hide, sit down, read, smoke and waste your time, the time they are paid for. That too is theft.

Most veterinarians simply do not think about the possible ways in which practice theft can occur. After the event they kick themselves and ask 'why didn't I realise how much lazy staff members are costing me? 'why didn't we establish better control over the petty cash?, or 'why didn't someone force me to bank daily or reconcile statements every month?"

Establish and enforce realistic control measures to reduce the risk and build a reputation in your practice that you will be very tough over dishonesty.

Theft of accounts owing can be made very simply by a staff member on behalf of a friend. A dishonest employee can make unauthorised entries in the adjustments, discounts, or returned fees area of the client's account on a pegboard or computer system. As a safeguard, review all returns, payments and discount adjustments daily or pick out record cards or computer records at random to be sure that all transactions have been properly recorded.

The best long term way of reducing theft is to be careful in recruiting. Follow up references by telephone. Previous employers may reveal by what they say or how they say it that there is some doubt about an employees honesty, a doubt which they would probably not reveal in writing.

If you suspect that theft or fraud may have already taken place.

- immediately seek the advice of your accountant and lawyer.
- always maintain a detailed inventory of equipment.
- restrict authority for ordering stock or equipment to specific named individuals.
- walk around the practice regularly, talk to your staff, ask them questions, open all the books and records from time to time and get into the habit of making random checks on all documentary procedures.

To maintain a good system of internal control you need to be more resourceful than the individual who may be stealing from you. Seek advice and design and implement a control system that will suit your practice requirements.

We don't want to overplay the problem. Very many practices have functioned for many years without a hint of dishonesty on the part of staff, clients or colleagues. Be in no doubt however that some practice owners have learned the hard way that internal practice security and control is as important a management task as any other.

If you do discover fraud, theft or dishonesty in the practice be very careful about accusing an individual. You should most certainly seek professional advice before you take any action concerning the staff member involved.

Selecting an Accountant

Many books on management will offer advice about selecting legal, financial, investment, insurance and other advisers to management. It may be opportune however, to make some suggestions about the selection of a practice accountant. Many veterinarians employ accountancy firms which simply act as expensive bookkeepers. They prepare the financial accounts, offer some tax advice and negotiate if necessary with the tax authorities. We believe that a more appropriate service should include advice in respect of practice performance, management accounts, practice valuation, buy-sell agreements, partnership negotiations, conducting feasibility studies for equipment acquisition, leasing versus buying decisions, investment, financial planning and a host of other matters. If this is the sort of service you seek, choose an accountant and a firm that can understand your individual needs as well as the needs of your business. Do not choose a firm that is too small or you may find that in the event of sickness or death of the principal that there is a lack of continuity. Some veterinarians would not choose a firm that is too large since the level of service, degree of expertise available and potential cost may be beyond that required by the practice.

Ask how fees are determined and to what extent the individuals who will be advising you have knowledge and experience of dealing with veterinary practice. We believe that some experience within the profession of veterinary medicine is critical. Enquire about the availability of partners and key personnel in the firm. There may be occasions when you will need the judgment, wisdom and experience of a more established partner in a firm or an individual who has particular knowledge and experience of the topic of concern at the time. One of the main purposes of engaging an accounting firm is to gain access to appropriate areas of expertise so that as the need arises you are in a position to make informed and intelligent practice investment and other decisions. Veterinarians in practice preach to their clients the wisdom of investing in professional veterinary advice. If you believe that to be true you will also accept the sense of investing your own or your practice resources in sound professional legal, accountancy or other advice.

Make some enquiries about the firms understanding of the veterinary profession with its particular business strengths and weaknesses. Ask how many veterinary practice clients are on their books, how they intend to maintain their current knowledge of veterinary business and other problems and whether they subscribe to periodicals dealing with such matters. Don't be penny wise and pound foolish. If sound advice, an ability to communicate, business judgement and professional acumen and integrity are your objectives, choose a firm with a vision beyond a financial statement and be prepared to pay for their services.

8

Computerisation

The Necessity and the Practice

The use of micro-processors in business has evolved from an interesting luxury to a present day necessity. In the 1970s many companies offered access to micro-processing systems. Many of the available systems were either too small for serious business application or demanded such a knowledge of electronics and computer technology that the typical small business person was completely intimidated.

IBM established a standard for a disk operating system and a path for growth that literally changed the mode of business. The dramatic changes in micro-processing have been of immense benefit for the professions. Commerce and industry and the medical based professions have been able to streamline costs, document clinical and other records, and store and manage data much more effectively and efficiently than ever before. The veterinary profession was amongst the first professions to see the opportunity and develop applications to help its members to cope with the growing burden of paperwork.

Over a period of a few years, 'stone-age' accounting and recording tools were replaced by the electronic-age equivalent. In most developed countries there is now a variety of 'value added' veterinary vendors who offer customised software that meets the specific needs of small animal, large animal, emergency clinic and specialty practices. The evolution of the software has developed to such a point that many companies are prepared to customise additional software segments to meet the particular needs of any practice.

Recent developments have greatly enhanced the 'user-friendly' attributes of computer hardware. New means have been found to pack more memory into smaller units of silicon with a quicker response time and the speed and power of micro-processing continues to grow logarithmically. Veterinarians have found that the equipment they purchase is outdated almost by the time the boxes are open and the computers are installed. As newer, better, quicker and more user friendly products are developed, older equipment has become obsolete. Fully functioning computer equipment has been discarded simply because the micro-processing speed was inadequate to meet the needs of software for other equipment available. Veterinarians who seem to be happy to retain aged cages, X-ray machines, autoclaves and other professional equipment seem to be very willing to upgrade computer equipment every two to three years.

The evolution of computerisation has however left its toll. There are a number of practice owners who are disinclined to computerise their practices because they have been badly let down by previous equipment or software suppliers. It is not uncommon to find a practice with expensive, space consuming, antiquated computer hardware afforded the status of a museum piece sitting in the corner of the practice principal's office.

Fortunately, the situation continues to improve dramatically. Multiple megabyte storage and memory processing capability have made the availability of easy to understand software a reality. Software companies have realised that the once arcane and unintelligible documentation traditionally associated with veterinary computer packages is simply not acceptable. Customers and veterinarians are extremely demanding. Any veterinary vendor who hopes to stay competitive and solvent has been forced to recognise the necessity of providing complete documentation and instructions. The need for clear and uncluttered training for every staff member is a critical part of the negotiation process between the practice owner or manager and the computer company representative. Video tapes, multi-colour manuals, competent sales representatives who actually know their systems and call free telephone lines are becoming standard for vendors offering software to the profession.

Too many software companies, however, still mislead potential customers by promising software programme features before they are actually available. This practice is known as 'promiseware'. Prudent purchasers should never decide to buy a computer system based on the features which are promised but which do not yet exist. The intentions may be sincere but inevitable delays, technological incapabilities, vendor budgets and programmer confidence all too often result in the timescale for 'promiseware' gestation to be overtaken by events. In the computer industry, a promise is merely a dream. A promise fulfilled is called a release.

The Return on Your Investment

Veterinarians have learned over the years that the purchase of a practice asset without an expectation of a monetary return on the investment can result in a severe financial strain on the practice. Every professional wants to acquire toys. Diagnostic instruments, surgical equipment, instruments and communications equipment have been purchased by veterinarians for many years with the financial reality being an afterthought. Computerisation cannot be purchased in the same manner. The casual and ill conceived acquisition of a computer system will not only result in a lost investment but untold stress, confusion and disappointment for the staff.

The installation of a modern computer system is most certainly not a simple turn-key proposition, contrary to popular opinion. Computerisation demands the preparation of a well thought out system specification for your practice. You will need to modify, adapt or discard many of the existing systems for recording and retrieving data and however smooth the process may be, it will take a substantial investment of your time and that of your staff to implement the new procedures. Financial projections will need to incorporate the costs of that investment and you must satisfy yourself that it will result in a positive financial return in the short term. Your investment in a computer system must be designed to pay for itself immediately it is operational.

If you are planning to purchase anything other than a single user system you should expect and demand that it will be operational within three months of delivery. If you anticipate a three month time scale you should not be surprised if the timetable is doubled or even tripled.

Your computer system can be a profitable investment by generating significant additional practice revenue and transaction volume. It will implement fee increases immediately and without error while ensuring that every single service provided by the practice and every single product used, dispensed or sold is charged for accurately and immediately.

Financial efficiency and improved staff productivity are important benefits of an effective computerised accounting and recording system in veterinary practice. The biggest contribution to enhance profitability is the ability to market the practice and the services it offers in a much more sophisticated and effective way.

A word processing programme for example, linked to the client database will enable a practice to add targeted messages for specific clients on receipts, invoices and statements. It will also prepare individual mailmerge letters to specific clients, client groups or owners of specific animal or patient groups with particular clinical problems or propensities. The computers contribution to the implementation of your marketing plan is limited only by your willingness to invest the time necessary to understand the market in which the practice operates and to target the particular clients or potential clients which you wish to contact.

Your computer must earn its keep. Let us look more closely at various situations to see how a computer can help you generate more practice income.

Cash Receipts

The flow of cash into a practice is its life blood. If a business is to survive it must generate cash. Profit is important. But unless it is quickly converted into cash, profit becomes simply an interesting financial entry which will be eventually written off. A computerised accounting system will help your practice to achieve that conversion.

In its simplest form a computer can be used as a cash receipt system for a small animal practice. The consulting veterinarian can check on screen or on a printout client and patient details. This could include the account history and any unpaid balances outstanding. After the consultation the veterinarian or the receptionist will record details of the treatment and services rendered and some systems enable memos to be passed between the clinician and receptionist to ensure that an appropriate further appointment is made. The receptionist can then reinforce the need for the specific treatment or follow up recommendations made by the consulting veterinarian.

A number of methods are used in veterinary practice for keying clinical and financial data into the client/patient database. In many practices in the United States, for example, the consulting veterinarian completes a worksheet which itemises the services rendered, procedures performed and stock items dispensed. The worksheet is generally sequentially numbered so that the practice has control over how they are recorded on the computer system. The client or veterinarian returns the worksheet to the front desk where the receptionist keys in the data. A fee schedule has already been incorporated into the program memory and pricing is automatic and consistent. Many large animal and equine practices use the same procedure. Worksheets are completed immediately. If the service has been completed on the farm then computer entries are keyed in as soon as the veterinarian returns to the practice.

Consistency in fee setting has important advantages for the practice. It helps to overcome the tendency for veterinarians, employers and employees, to reduce fees for emotional reasons. Fee increases can be updated instantaneously and most systems will offer either across the board percentage increase or selective increases for particular procedures or stock items. Many programs also offer the option of linking particular procedures with the stock items associated with that treatment. This ensures that the receptionist or consulting veterinarian who keys in the particular clinical service is assured that the disposable items, injections and other medication associated with the service are priced and that the appropriate stock items are deleted from the inventory.

Many other practices, particularly in the UK, have computer terminals in the consulting room, laboratory, preparation or treatment room or the hospital so that the veterinarian or nurse is able to monitor clinical and financial history and key in clinical and other data immediately.

While this system reduces duplication of effort it does enable the consulting veterinarian to use the computer capability to modify (reduce) the fee if he chooses to do so. For this reason, many practices which have the capability for terminal input in the consulting room to enable the consulting veterinarian to monitor the previous history, still insist that data entry is carried out at reception. The worksheet becomes a separate document that can be monitored by the receptionist to spot any errors or service omissions. It can also be used as a checklist before the clinician sees the patient. In this approach the reception staff can indicate in advance on the worksheet that the client has, for example, requested a particular service.

There is no 'right' or 'wrong' system and much will depend on the management style and routine appropriate to the particular practice and as determined by the veterinarian, manager or hospital director responsible.

A computerised cash receipt system will automatically analyse the mode of payment e.g. by cash, cheque, credit or charge card. This is very helpful when submitting cheques and credit card receipts for payment to the bank and facilitates the day end task of reconciling cash, cheque and credit card slips in the till with the summary printout of receipts for the day.

The difference between fees earned and cash received is posted to the individual clients financial record and to the debtors list. The system allows the practice to maintain a much firmer credit control procedure. Clerical errors are eliminated and no longer will one client's account be mischarged for the services that another client, with a similar name, has received. The client database can usually be searched by name or code number and client and patient details can be checked thoroughly by the reception staff prior to the consultation. In this way the database details are kept up to date.

Once the data has been posted, a variety of management reports, reports that would normally take many hours to prepare, are available with a key stroke. They will include a daily analysis of fees charged, case volume and receipts and monthly summaries with an aged accounts receivable (aged debtors) list.

Revenue analysis can usually be predetermined by the practice manager or director and may include revenue classification by patient species, procedure, consulting veterinarian or any other chosen parameter. Such reports can form the basis for monitoring staff productivity and a variety of performance based payment schemes.

Some sophisticated systems will co-ordinate salary, fringe benefit and payroll tax details for each employee veterinarian and calculate a gross profit contribution earned by that individual for the practice on a daily basis.

The computer software enables prompt interest charges to be added to outstanding accounts and lists of those clients with outstanding accounts can be prepared at will. This enables the appropriate follow up policy to be pursued vigorously. Interest and service fees which can be charged will depend on the law as it applies in the country concerned. It is customary for many practices to charge a billing fee (an account fee) or an interest charge of at least one and a half percent per month, whichever is the greater. Some practices charge both a billing fee and an interest rate. The law in some countries will not allow professional practices to assess interest for billing charges without previous notification to the client and veterinarians are advised to seek legal advice in this respect if they are in any doubt.

Your Precious Database

Recently designed software programs for veterinary practice have all incorporated a relational database that permits veterinarians far greater latitude in searching client and patient information for marketing purposes. Every time a particular client telephones or visits the practice the appropriate database record should be called up to enable a check to be made that all details are up to date. The search possibilities are endless. It is possible to identify, list with address and telephone numbers and prepare mailmerge letters for a number of client or patient groups.

The database is particularly useful to identify clients who may not have made contact with the practice for some time so that a telephone call or letter may be used to enquire as to the general health of the pet. More commonly, database information is used to establish and monitor a number of clinical recall and follow up reminders for those patients with specific ongoing clinical conditions. This capability in a non-computerised system would be virtually impossible because of the time it would take to review individual client records to glean the same information.

Eighty percent of your practice income will be generated by 20% of your clients and we believe that you should spend a great deal of your time nurturing and supporting that 20%. That is not to say that the 80% should be neglected — in fact you should do everything you can to convert them to potential '20 percenters' to replace those who die, do not replace their pet animals or who leave the locality.

Watching over your best clients is one of the best practice tips ever afforded to any professional. Generally speaking too much time is spent trying to acquire new clients to sustain growth. Veterinarians spend too little time trying to meet the needs of faithful, loyal clients who have stayed with the practice for many years. A computer system will help to identify the 20% — your most valuable clients. The phrase 'thank you' is a powerful marketing tool. Practice principals should allocate some of their practice day to renewing contact with those long term clients who have played a major contribution to practice growth.

When purchasing a computer system ensure that it has the capability for a number of search options which may not be related to routine management reporting. Such an option will enable veterinarian to be creative and be able to 'tag' particular clients or client groups for a particular reason. Suppose you were able to identify for example, particular clients who have always had a keen interest in their animal's health and have always settled their accounts promptly but who have been badly hit by the impact of economic recession locally. You would surely want to encourage such pet owners to continue to seek and take veterinary advice even if payment will be delayed? You may decide to offer discounts or long term payment schedules without interest to such clients because you appreciate that the risk of possible non-payment is outweighed by the probability that the client will eventually pay and will remember the kindness that you extended during their financial difficulties. Do not forget that, within reason, a higher receivable balance (debtors) during a period of economic difficulty is preferable to losing a valued client. Your computer could be an invaluable tool in identifying, tagging and offering particular concessions to them without upsetting the normal accounting constraints.

Part of the specification for your proposed computer system should relate to such capabilities. Ask sales representatives to sit down with you to demonstrate the test data that they bring with them and then ask how you would select specific items of data for a relational database inquiry. Make sure that the programme will enable you to identify those clients who have spent the most money in your practice over a period of time. These are the clients that are worth continued attention. These are the clients who should contribute most to the success of the financial plan for your practice for the next two or three years.

Stock Control (Inventory)

Most veterinary software programs include a stock control module that should enable the practice to maintain a perpetual record of medicines and other items in stock. The system will record increased stock levels resulting from purchases and depleted stock resulting from sales. For reasons which we have already identified however, the stock list determined by the computer may not equate with the stock on the shelf. Many practices do not maintain perpetual stock holding levels on computer because they regard the time and cost of keying in all the purchases

as being far greater than the benefit that can be derived. Other practices, on the other hand, do maintain stock levels on computer as a record-keeping measure for monitoring purchase levels for drugs and professional supplies over a period of time. The latter information can be valuable when negotiating advantageous pricing terms with suppliers.

Major discrepancies between actual stock levels and stock levels identified by the software program could indicate theft. Most veterinarians would agree, however, that a close watch on purchasing trends and the frequency that drugs are being ordered can be even more effective as part of an overall stock control system.

Accounts Payable and Purchase Ledger

A number of options are possible. Many veterinary practices use computer based software for clinical and financial records and to prepare sales ledger data while maintaining a simple handwritten purchase ledger. With this software they can monitor standing orders, direct debit payments, cheque and petty cash payments and allocate costs to a number of standard cost headings. Others use standard accounting packages that will summarise payments and reconcile bank statements. A few use software programs which are fully integrated and incorporate a stock control component.

Much will depend on the precise needs of the management accounting system required for the particular practice. We recommend that the issues are discussed with the practice accountant and that the likely training and staff costs are considered in addition to the direct costs of the appropriate software requirement.

There are a number of other issues which you will need to consider in some depth in the preparation of a specification for your computer installation. They include:

General Ledger and Financial Accounting

In recent years veterinary practice owners and managers, and their accountants, have realised that there is a need to standardise data so that meaningful comparisons can be made. The

American Animal Hospital Association has published a standardised chart of accounts which, together with an appropriate computer based accounting system, enables practices to post receipts and payments directly into a general ledger system using appropriate nominal codes for subsequent analysis. There are many such accounting software systems, with varying levels of complexity on the market. They all have the advantage of being able to prepare monthly profit and loss statements, balance sheets and budget updates based on cost and revenue headings determined by the practice owner. Some maintenance is required when new accounts are added or when different statements are needed, but the routine report format once established remains constant and can be run automatically at the end of each month.

One of the major benefits of a computer system is that a reliable keyboard operator who may not have the sophisticated skills and knowledge of a trained bookkeeper, is able to prepare a fairly accurate cash basis financial statement for management use on a monthly basis. This does not reduce the need for the services of an accountant but it does mean that, instead of providing a costly book-keeping service, his advice can be sought for his judgement and business knowledge as well as financial and tax acumen.

With appropriate advice from your Chartered Accountant or CPA, an office or practice manager should have the necessary knowledge and ability either to input data themselves or to assign the task to an accounts clerk or other employee. If the veterinarian is prepared to invest in planning and setting up an electronic general ledger system with the help of the practice accountant, an in-house employee can certainly be trained to use it. If your accountant is unwilling to help, find a new accountant. Most progressive accounting firms will not only help you but they should already have encouraged you to invest in computer technology.

It may be sensible to install a general ledger system in the practice which is compatible with your accountant's system. If you utilise the same general ledger system as your accountant, it may be possible to transmit data either by floppy disk or by modem to the accountant's office. This arrangement should eliminate at least some of the accounting fees because it will reduce the necessity of keying in some data on more than one occasion.

Printing Options

Be aware of the many options. Ensure that the answers to a number of questions are clear before you make any purchase decisions. Can the system operate with a laser printer? Can the typeface for the specific programs be changed either by cartridge in a laser printer or by specific software drivers that will interact with the computer software? Can the veterinary software package be run in Windows? (Microsoft Corporation reg) to enable financial data derived from the veterinary software package to be cut and pasted to a graphics program for presentation? Can the system add messages? Is it completely interchangeable with either your present word processing program or its own word processing program, to enable staff to include specific clinical messages or reminders on invoices or receipts for the clients attention? Remember that the paperwork produced by your practice for clients must reflect the overall image you wish to project for every single aspect of practice activity. If you seek an image for high quality professional standards of service, do not spoil the impact with poor quality printing or paperwork. Matrix printers are commonplace but they are noisy and you may decide to invest in the enhanced graphics output capabilities of a laser printer.

Graphics — Spreadsheet Capabilities

Veterinarians are generally becoming aware of the value of a number of software tools of which word processing and spreadsheet capabilities are perhaps the most common. Spreadsheet programmes such as the ever popular Lotus 123, Borlands, Quattro, Microsoft, Excel and a number of others, can be used to illustrate financial and other trends in a variety of graphic forms in addition to their ability to perform 'what if?' calculations in an instant. Data imported from 'value added' veterinary software programs can be analysed and summarised to prepare budgets and cash flow forecasts and to monitor operational performance in a variety of ways in a spreadsheet programme.

Spreadsheets can also be extremely valuable in planning the financial costs of a number of options for performance based salary packages for employees. They are also valuable for calculating base salaries relating to individual gross and bonus payments for particular employees.

One of the features to be incorporated in the specification of a computer system for your practice would be a facility for transporting data from the veterinary package to a spreadsheet program. You may also wish to consider the possibility of transferring data from the 'value added' program to off the shelf data management programs such as D-BASE IV and Paradox. Translation utilities are available with some software programs to transfer selected data directly into alternative data management programs. Producers of veterinary software packages will increasingly need to incorporate translation utilities to enable data to be exported to a number of 'off the shelf' software programs.

Word Processing

Stand alone word processing systems and desktop publishing programs linked with laser printers have become increasingly popular and user friendly over the last three years. Sophisticated desktop publishing programs offer an enormous range of type style, font and graphic options but they require a significant additional investment in staff training. Some of the more sophisticated stand alone programs are easier to use and may be totally adequate to satisfy the practice requirements for well designed newsletters and other documentation. Word processing requirements will need to be considered and incorporated in the practice computer specification.

Electronic Communication

A fax machine is easy to operate and requires very little specialised skill. More and more veterinary practices are using fax equipment to order stock, receive laboratory reports, transmit clinical histories to specialists and for many other professional and business purposes. Modem facilities too are becoming increasingly valuable in veterinary practice. Many practices are linked by modem, for example, to the suppliers of their veterinary practice computer packages. A modem is simply a device that permits one computer to talk to another computer. With software programs such as Carbon Copy Plus, a software support operator at a remote site can operate the practice computer. Similarly a 'guest' computer at a practice ten miles away can call up a 'host' computer and gain access to all of its records, files and software programmes. This is a different and distinct facility from the mere ability to transfer files between two computers.

The potential for instant access to information, knowledge and expertise by electronic means is enormous. It is only limited by economic factors and the imagination of those who have and those who wish to have the information available.

Data Storage

The hard disk is the essential heart of any computer based data handling system for serious business purposes. Memory requirements are prodigious. A few years ago a ten megabyte system was considered state of the art. Now, veterinarians routinely require a computer system with a minimum of 320 megabytes of storage. By adding additional hard disks or larger hard disks, a practice can increase its storage capability to well past a gigabyte of data.

Other technology which will continue to develop and which will have an impact on the information requirements of veterinary practice includes CD-ROM technology. The ability to pack data very densely in disks very similar to CD records and then access it through laser technology is at an early stage of practical development for veterinary practice. We believe the future role of such technology within the profession to be very exciting.

CD technology using equipment which will read and write data on CD disc will enable practices to gain immediate access to written, graphic, sound and video/film information and will also be used as a reliable method of data backup within veterinary practice. CD technology will also be used in the production and development of equipment used in house to inform and instruct clients about the clinical conditions affecting their animals and the diagnostic, medical and other procedures which are recommended.

System Security

Once you are computerised you are also vulnerable. It may be unlikely but it is certainly possible that a dishonest employee could access your data file system and copy it through the backup utility. They could, for example, selectively make copies of specific files for their own use. That is theft. You should be aware of the possibilities and consider at the outset the need to restrict access to your computer system at certain levels by means of a password system. In spite of modern technology your system is also vulnerable to unexpected and often unexplained breakdown. You must insist that every member of the practice maintains the strict discipline associated with the need for a regular backup system, with at least one backup level of tapes kept away from the practice premises in case of a disaster.

Buy from an Established Vendor

In the early days of computerisation, veterinary software vendors came and went as rapidly as the technological changes in hardware. Whenever you invest in a computer system there is an element of risk relating to the reliability of the software programs you use as well as the processors, disk drives, backup systems, terminals, printers and all the other hardware items. There is also some risk that the system you purchase may be obsolete within a relatively short time or that the memory you specified at the outset is inadequate within a few months. You may find that the level of training and maintenance which seemed appropriate when you signed the contract, is now just not good enough. If you want to eliminate all the risks you will never invest in a computer. If however, you want to keep the risks to a minimum, you should certainly purchase from a reliable and established supplier.

You could, for example, make enquiries about the financial viability of the company concerned.

In the United States for example, you could seek a credit report from Dun & Bradstreet to ensure as far as possible that imminent bankruptcy is unlikely and that the company has the financial capability to stay afloat at least during the warranty period but hopefully well beyond that.

Seeking a financial health-check is only one of the steps you should take in evaluating the vendor with which you plan to do business. Ask for the names of plenty of practice owners who have already purchased the system so that you can talk to them about it. Ask them if it has fulfilled their expectations. Make sure that the individuals you approach do not have a vested interest in the vendor company. Ask how long they have used the system and how many keyboard and other operators they have changed since it was installed. Ask whether the vendor has been helpful and willing to help to resolve any problems. Ask about the quality of training, support and documentation. Enquire as to the support time for repair of equipment and ask whether the vendor will provide substitute equipment while the practice's equipment is being repaired.

Make sure that the contract you are asked to sign is acceptable. That means reading and understanding it. Specifically, the license to use the software must be transferable to a third party if you were, for example, to sell the practice. Also ask whether the system could be sold to another veterinarian with the same warranty if you were to update your system and purchase from an alternative vendor. Don't rely upon verbal representations from the salesman. Ensure that the answers to such important questions are provided in writing by an authorised officer of the vendor company.

Don't rely exclusively on the word of the sales representative unless you have also talked with the owners of a few current installations. Sometimes veterinary computer companies provide superb service, excellent hardware, develop a fantastic reputation and grow dramatically. As their profit margins increase their attention to individual customers has been known to decline. When that happens, the company may attempt to ride on its earlier reputation. You may talk to a user who has had wonderful experiences with the system some years ago while discussion with a more recent purchaser may reveal a different story.

Remember that you may be dealing with a particular salesman on a long-term basis. What was your first impression of him? Ensure that the sales representations are based upon the merits of the system they are selling and not on the deficiencies of the competition.

Be Wary of Extra Features

It is not unreasonable for veterinary computer representatives to stress the importance of a range of dazzling features which are not available on other systems. It is not sensible however for a potential purchaser to be seduced by those features which may add considerably to the cost of the system but which may never be used. The exciting extras, the endless possibilities for management reports and the 'promiseware' round the corner can be very attractive - and very expensive. Our advice is always to spend a good deal of time and effort in preparing a required specification for your practice before you go out into the marketplace.

When the time comes to make specific enquiries to the company salesman, insist that they demon-strate the feature to which you refer or to point it out in the documentation. Note exactly when and how it may be used. Oral representations are difficult to prove if the computer system is faulty. By that time the salesman may have left the company or may deny that the claim was ever made if there are no witnesses or documentation to confirm what you say.

Very many exotic computer features are rarely used. This is particularly true for stock (inventory) control systems. In our experience computerised stock control systems in veterinary practice are excellent for maintaining a stock database with suppliers, pack sizes, prices and so on. They are also valuable for monitoring stock usage but are not to be trusted for preparing stock order lists. The problems lie not in the hardware or software but simply because the large volume of relatively small stock items involves such a lot of slippage, spillage and waste that the actual stock holding on the shelf rarely matches the stock holding determined by the computer.

Summary

Selection of the appropriate computerised system for any particular veterinary practice will depend on the practice owners understanding of the needs of the business for data storage and retrieval, on an awareness of the ways in which computer hardware and software can satisfy those needs and of the practices ability to afford the investment required. Electronic management of data requires stewardship and tending. Selection of the appropriate system is only the first stage. Unless the practice owner, director or manager is prepared to be actively involved in planning and implementing the changeover from a manual to a computer based system, the investment will be wasted.

The vendors of 'value added' systems may know their product but they don't know your practice. You must ensure that you have considered every single clerical task under your existing system and clarified whether it will be replaced by or modified as a result of the new system. Some management consultants are able to assist veterinarians with this task. It is still important for the veterinarian who does purchase a substantial computer system to devote sufficient resources and management time to keep the system current. You should expect to incur substantial reinvestment in your computer installation every three years.

If you have a computer already, spend some time and reread the documentation. You will be surprised by how much more you will know and understand about your own system and what additional benefits you can derive from it. If you do not have a computer yet try to become computer literate. Explore the possibilities and opportunities available as soon as possible. You could lose out if your practice does not make use of the many advantages of computer technology as we approach the remaining years of the 20th Century.

9

Valuing A Veterinary Practice

Valuation of any asset depends on the circumstances and on the objectives of the parties involved. The validity of a final valuation can only be determined when agreement is reached between a willing vendor and a capable purchaser to transfer the title of the asset at the price agreed.

The objective of a practice valuation is usually to establish a fair and equitable price to enable the practice owner, the vendor, to negotiate an agreement with a potential purchaser. If a fair and equitable price is known, the vendor can then establish a negotiating position armed with the knowledge of relative fair worth.

It is an increasingly common practice for purchasers and vendors to agree in advance to seek the views of an independent specialist adviser to determine the value of each of the practice assets and to accept jointly, his impartial conclusions. Frequently, the vendor and the purchaser have sufficient and equal confidence in the impartiality and competence of the specialist to award such a degree of trust in one person's opinion. In such circumstances both parties benefit by limiting the number of advisers and specialists that become involved in the sales transaction.

The purchaser and vendor will still engage separate legal representation to advise them in respect of their rights and obligations in the contractual arrangement. The professional valuer may be appointed to offer suggestions to both the vendor and the purchaser. Assuming that he is not engaged on an advocacy basis, the valuer must take every effort to provide the same information to vendor and purchaser and their professional advisers.

As idealistic and simple as the idea of one valuation adviser may be, circumstances may determine otherwise. If the valuation advisers are engaged on an advocacy basis, their respective opinions of value and the methodology used should not be different than when engaged on an independent basis. However, the information they offer and any tactical suggestions they may make in the negotiation process will be restricted solely to the interests of their particular clients.

Practice purchase/sale situations frequently involve a great deal of negotiation to ensure that buyer and seller are both satisfied signatories to the agreement. Equally as important however, interested third parties like bank managers, executors and so on, may also need to be convinced that the best possible price was agreed for their respective clients in the negotiation process. They may like to see a little blood spilt to be ensured that the final purchase price is realistic. Please don't forget however, that the price exacted from the blood letting may be very expensive. You should consider the alternative, a civilised discussion between the vendor, purchaser, advisers and interested third parties to strike a less costly and more satisfactory agreement for all concerned.

For an independent practice valuation to be useful, the interests of both parties must be carried out from the point of reference of a third party investor taking a detached, unemotional, view of the proposed transaction.

In any practice valuation, a large number of intangible factors will enhance or reduce the value of the practice in the eyes of the owner or a possible purchaser. Unquantifiable strengths or weaknesses not included in the formal valuation model must however be addressed. Potential growth because of an exciting demographic location, prior neglect of the practice clientele, less than professional standards of veterinary medicine and lack of modern equipment are all factors which may not show up in any documentation but may significantly affect the success of the practice enterprise. These intangible factors will have an important part to play in the desirable and inevitable negotiation which will ultimately determine the price agreed.

A credible and realistic valuation must be based on a thorough understanding of the practice. Simple rules of thumb to determine a valuation are unlikely to satisfy the needs of both parties and are not likely to be workable. Most vendors and purchasers are advised to seek the advice of an independent valuer experienced in such matters.

As a starting point, the vendor must provide a valuer with all the information required to establish a realistic valuation, including reliable and accurate financial and management accounting data, complete lists of equipment, fixtures and fittings with a full description of their condition, aged accounts and a complete list of all liabilities, stated and unstated. Other practice assets such as currency and currency equivalents, deposits, prepaid expenses, investments and so on, must also be revealed to the valuer. Because the basis of accounting may not include all of these assets at their actual cash value, the vendor must not assume that the accountant's financial statements are adequate or complete.

A formal valuation is not limited to the purchase and sale of a veterinary practice. Valuation is also required for a partnership purchase, in the retirement of a senior partner, in divorce proceedings and, on an annual basis, as an essential element in practice management.

Valuation Methods

Income Method

If the asset produces an income (e.g. a rented building or business), the value can be based on the return achieved. By capitalising the expected revenue at a reasonable return on investment over a long term basis, the value of the asset is determined by the quantification of the net expected earnings it generates. The percentage return on investment required is affected by the relative risk which the asset has in generating income over a number of years.

Delivery of goodwill is a critical element to consider in relying upon the income method of valuation. Circumstances may arise that could place the expectation of future income in jeopardy. For example, the vendor may have every intention of setting up in competition in close proximity to the practice that is available for sale. Because the vendor has access to all of the client lists and patient records in the practice to be sold, he may have every opportunity to encourage his clients to frequent his new veterinary practice. The potential purchaser of such a practice would be foolish to invest in goodwill which the vendor has no intention of delivering. Such examples may be rare, but purchasers are advised to incorporate a restrictive covenant in the purchase contract, drafted by their legal adviser, to protect their rights in this respect.

Another example would be a practice where the principal has died and the estate has not arranged for a relief veterinarian to provide professional cover until a new owner can be found. In the intervening period, many clients could have found alternative services and the value of the practice would decline as a result.

When a cloud looms over the delivery of goodwill, a choice exists:

- The capitalisation rate can be adjusted downward to reflect the greater risk.
- Earnings can be reduced to identify the specific area of delivery doubt.
- A contingent purchase price can be arranged to let the future potential determine the ultimate price paid.

In circumstances where significant doubts exist, the fears of the purchaser as to what is really being purchased can be mitigated to some extent with a contingent purchase price to quantify the goodwill. Usually a time period of three to five years is selected as the contingent purchase period. The new purchaser operates the practice for the agreed period. At the conclusion of the period, the practice value is recalculated based upon the capitalisation of net earnings at that time. A purchase price is calculated and agreed, and the price is then discounted back to the currency equivalent at the date of the original transaction. The discount rate is usually agreed by the parties as part of the documentation of the contingent purchase agreement. Payments of principal and interest are recalculated and the amortisation is carried forward to the date of calculation. There are a number of potential difficulties with such an arrangement however, and the contingent purchase agreement solution is not appropriate for all practice situations. It does merit consideration however, especially if the negotiation process is breaking down in a series of 'what if's'.

Market Method

The market method assesses the value of an asset based on a comparison with the recent sale of a similar asset. This is a useful approach when valuing property which is not used for revenue purposes. To some extent valuation here depends on scarcity value. The market method cannot be used reliably to value the goodwill of a veterinary practice. Attempts to express the value of goodwill on a simple percentage of gross receipts are equally unreliable. An example of how the market method would be used most characteristically, is in the purchase and sale of a personal residence.

Cost Method

The cost method depends on identifying the replacement cost of the asset and reducing it by a depreciation factor representing relative wear, tear, and obsolescence to arrive at the actual cash value of the asset. Variations of the cost method include historical financial statement cost, financial statement book value and tax basis book value.

It is often sensible to approach a particular valuation using more than one of the methods we have outlined. A comparative analysis of the values achieved as the result of differing approaches can assist in assessing a value which can be defended if necessary in tough negotiation. Since a veterinary practice is composed of a number of assets, both tangible and intangible, a number of valuation methods will need to be utilised. An experience veterinary practice valuer will assess the appropriate method to use.

For example, a professional real estate appraiser might value a residential rental property in a number of ways. The market method of valuation would take into account the sale prices of properties similar to that for sale and which have recently been sold in the neighbourhood.

The cost method of valuation would be to determine a current rebuilding cost for the property, less a sum representing fair wear and tear plus the value of the land.

The income method would be based on an assumption that the property would be rented to a third party at a fair market value. The valuer would determine the total rent which could be expected, less an appropriate sum to cover interest, insurance and other expenses to determine an estimated profit. The profit is then capitalised based on a reasonable return on investment.

The examples we have quoted simply illustrate that a number of methods may be used to value any asset and the appropriate approach for any specific item will depend on the particular circumstances and conditions which prevail.

Valuing Your Practice

Practice Property

The value of your practice property should be assessed by a competent qualified professional real estate valuer who has a knowledge of the property market in your locality. Under some circumstances, for example in partnership purchase or sale negotiations, the parties will agree to accept the recommendation of a well respected local valuer. On other occasions however, the parties prefer to seek independent advice. It is not uncommon to find a significant difference between the two values on such occasions.

Be clear about the specific instructions which are given to the valuer as a basis for valuation. Much will depend on the current state of the market locally but an open market value based on vacant possession is likely to be the basis chosen by a practice vendor, particularly if an enhanced price could be achieved if the sale of the property was not necessarily restricted to a veterinary buyer.

Instruments and Equipment

Veterinary practices invest in a wide range of equipment as well as specialist and general surgical and other instruments. Individual items will range from motor vehicles to radiographic equipment, from suture needles to operating lamps and from filing cabinets to computers.

The market method is usually used to assess large value professional and office equipment, furniture and fixtures and electronic cash registers and computers. For extremely significant tangible individual property, an expert appraisal of the specific equipment may be needed. For example, the radiographic equipment may be appraised by a representative of the manufacturer who is very familiar with the market for used apparatus of this type.

For less valuable equipment and furniture, the replacement value for a comparable asset is used as a starting point and is then depreciated on the basis of its likely residual life. The condition of the asset is assessed by the purchaser and the vendor. Hopefully, both can reasonably agree as to the remaining useful life and the quality and condition of the assets. In most cases buyers and sellers are able to agree an overall valuation for such assets without much difficulty.

In the UK there is a generally accepted protocol to value items which are in excellent condition and which are less than (say) six months old at around 75% of replacement value. Items which are older than six months and which have been subject to some normal wear and tear would be discounted by around 50%. Older items would be valued at anything between 25% and nil depending on their age and condition.

In the United States, professional equipment would be valued at a higher percentage than furniture and fixtures. Some veterinary equipment in excellent condition, which is not subject to technological obsolescence such as stainless steel cages, can be valued from 85% to 95% of replacement cost. Dependent upon the condition and age of the asset, medical equipment is usually valued at 70% to 90% of replacement cost. However, if the medical equipment is superseded by more up-to-date technology (such as laboratory diagnostic equipment) the value as a percentage of replacement cost could range from 50% to 85%. Furniture can range in worth, based upon condition and age, from 20% to 75% of replacement cost. Computer

equipment is subject to considerable discounted value because of technological updates. The percentage of replacement cost can range from 20% to 80%, but the age of the computer will have a much greater impact on its value than furniture or medical equipment of a similar age.

The valuation of practice vehicles, some office equipment and household items will all be based on market values and should not cause any difficulty between a genuine buyer and seller who are keen to reach a negotiated settlement. Large or expensive items will generally be subject to separate negotiation but smaller items may well be grouped and valued together so that a reasonable overall value can be agreed for the lot. This may include a number of individual items, some of which will be marginally overvalued and some undervalued.

As we stated above, care should be taken with computer systems. In many cases computer hardware older than two or three years has very little residual value unless it is capable of significant upgrading.

Software packages may also have a limited value and care should be taken by the purchaser to ensure that rights to utilise the software can be transferred to the purchaser and under what circumstances and at what cost upgrades can be provided. Caveat emptor must be the guide in the purchase of used computer hardware and software. Remember that the computer user is generally only licensed to utilise the software rather than own it. Permission must then be sought by the user to transfer the licence to the new owner of the equipment.

Value-added veterinary vendor software applications which are widely used in the United States and Canada have an option to ensure that the most current versions of the software are supplied to the practice through a software maintenance agreement. If the practice to be purchased has maintained this software maintenance agreement from the outset, the value of the software may be equivalent to its current list price. However, a precondition of valuing the software at list price is the continued existence of the software vendor without the prospect of bankruptcy. A purchaser of a veterinary practice should arrange for the vendor to obtain a letter of representation from the software vendor certifying that the purchaser will have the same successor rights as the present practice owner. If the practice to be purchased is incorporated, this representation letter may be unnecessary since the common stock of the practice entity is sold rather than the specific assets.

The important first step for the potential vendor (seller) of a veterinary practice is to draw up a comprehensive list of instruments and items of equipment with one column alongside to note the age and condition of the item, a second column for the estimated replacement cost and a third column to be used subsequently to estimate/calculate the asking price.

Drugs and Other Stock Items

Drugs and professional supplies are usually valued at current replacement cost. The normal approach is to prepare a comprehensive list of stock items in advance of the completion of the sale. On the day of completion, individual items are counted and valued on the basis of recent invoice or catalogue prices. The normal procedure is to exclude open bottles, boxes and packets and out of date stock. Dated stock items which are close to their expiration date will be discounted significantly, particularly if they are likely to be used infrequently. Other dated stock items which may be used quickly may, on the other hand, be valued at 100% of replacement price. Vendors in particular should be careful that the catalogues used to determine replacement costs are current. Some judgement will need to be made by the vendor as to the replacement value of a particular stock item which he was able to purchase at a significantly discounted rate, because of a particular bulk or other purchase deal.

We believe that honesty is the best policy. Negotiations between a genuine vendor and purchaser are unlikely to break down over a dispute over stock values. Both the vendor and purchaser must communicate any concerns they may have over the tallying of the drug and professional supply inventory early so that any misunderstandings can be identified and dealt with promptly.

The development of a variety of 'value added' veterinary computer software packages has resulted in a number of sophisticated electronic stock control systems. In theory they have the ability to generate up to date stock lists and order requirements at any time. In our view however, their greatest value is in monitoring stock usage and a physical stock take should be undertaken at least annually and certainly at the time of a sale. Even if the perpetual inventory record is reconciled to the annual physical inventory, we have found that a separate physical inventory should be taken for drugs and professional supplies at or near the transaction date for the sale of the practice.

Other Issues

Generally a purchase agreement will ensure that the vendor is responsible for all outstanding creditors at the time of the sale and that subsequent receipts from debtors are the property of the vendor. Occasionally, to overcome the practical difficulties of correctly allocating practice receipts after the sale, an agreement may be reached for the purchaser to pay an appropriate sum to buy the outstanding debtors (accounts receivable). The value to be placed on this figure is however arguable and a prudent purchaser will seek to discount it substantially before reaching such an agreement.

In large animal or mixed practices, the extent of the receivables may be so significant that a contingent purchase agreement is made as part of the purchase document. With this approach, an estimated value for the aged accounts receivable is included as a component part of the assets in the practice. A period of time, usually a year, is needed to determine the actual accounts receivable which are collected. Based upon the historical collection experience, the purchase price of the assets are then adjusted and recalculated. The parties thus value the aged accounts based on the sum actually collected, instead of speculating on the percentage of debtor assets which have ultimately been paid in previous years.

Some practice assets may not be included on the balance sheet. One such example is the value of the practice goodwill. Other such assets might include deposits, patents and rights of future income and computerised patient record systems.

Two elements exist for the patient record system — keypunch time and the intangible value of the client/patient for future generation of income. The input of patient and client records into the computer system takes time. Keypunch time is usually costed according to the estimated time taken to replicate the entire patient files in the value added veterinary vendor system and is subject to the level of detail involved.

The relative value of the keypunch time for patient records also depends on the reliability of the veterinary computer software system. Clearly it will be of much less value if the value added veterinary software vendor is no longer in existence. Major vendor software commands more respect, and the keypunch time needed to implement the system has more value if the software has commercial staying power. For this reason 'major player' software will permit a higher value to be placed on the keypunch time of the patient record system.

A favourable leasehold term provides an off-balance sheet asset since the cost to lease the premises is less than the market would dictate. In the late 1970s and early 1980s, a favourable lease was not uncommon. However, in the early 1990s some older leases may be regarded almost as a liability rather than an asset.

In an ideal situation, liabilities are all paid before the practice assets are transferred. However, the real world does not work that way. In establishing a fair value for the practice, a purchaser must ensure that all liabilities are identified as at the valuation date and the purchase price adjusted accordingly. The liabilities may all be identified in the financial statements, books and records of the practice but for those practices that run a cash basis of accounting, it may be difficult to identify them all.

Some liabilities such as accounts payable, accrued expenses, and some long-term financing arrangement (e.g. lease commitments) may not be included in the balance sheet. It is not unknown for example, for practices to include the value of leased assets in totalling total assets but forget

to identify the liability resulting from the stream of remaining lease payments which have been committed. Long-term lease commitments for specific property rentals must be considered in relationship to the current market value of the lease.

In the past it was a reasonable assumption that the cost of leased space would continue to rise and that a long-term lease would generate a valuable balance sheet asset. In many parts of the world, the value of leased space has however declined significantly. If the practice is committed to a long-term lease at a rate which is in excess of the current market rate for similar space at a similar location, a liability has been established and must be recognised by the vendor and by a purchaser. The present value of the lease commitment which exceeds a current fair market valuation is an unstated liability that must be accounted as an additional reduction in the value of the practice.

Care must be taken to include only the fair market value rental of the premises in calculating the net profit of the practice. If the lease payment is included at a value in excess of the fair market value rental in calculating goodwill, the present value of the lease must not be included as an unstated asset. Professional advice should be sought since, if considerable care is not taken, either goodwill will be understated or liabilities, to the extent of the present value of the excess lease, would be overstated.

Some liabilities may be personal to the vendor and may not be known accurately as at the date of valuation. Legal advice must be sought by the purchaser to ensure that the contract of purchase provides that they are not faced with an unexpected commitment some time after the contract has been signed, sealed and delivered.

Goodwill

Every profitable business is likely to have a value over and above the value of its net tangible assets. For convenience the difference between the two may be described as goodwill. The goodwill value for any particular business depends on the willingness of the vendor to sell at that price and the ability of a willing purchaser to pay for it.

The goodwill valuation will be affected by a wide range of variable factors but is related in some way to the profitability of the practice. Goodwill is usually quantified in terms capitalising the value of excess earnings. Excess earnings may be defined as a measure of true profit for the practice owner after deducting a realistic figure which represents the costs of his time invested in the business.

A number of external factors will have an impact on practice profitability and may therefore affect the goodwill valuation. They will include:

- A favourable location for the veterinary practice with good visibility unobstructed by other signs and pleasantly designed with appropriate landscaping.
- A fully operational ongoing concern with a high standard of accounting, clinical and client records.
- Adequate space with a workable traffic flow for clients, patients and staff.
- Planning approval as appropriate.
- Established for some time, good reputation and listed in telephone books, yellow pages and other directories.
- Low rate of client turnover.
- Appropriate mix of socio-economic groups and income levels in the catchment area of the practice.
- Good communications (road and public transport) to local areas of population.
- The existence of effective workable internal control systems to safeguard the collection of cash and the maintenance of an effective inventory control system.
- Employee loyalty to the practice and technical competence.

Your practice may have some or all of these attributes but unless they contribute to achieving significant levels of profit, the goodwill value will be limited.

A practice that has a good location, excellent clinical and business skills and ability, low client turnover, employee loyalty, an excellent reputation within the community and good data retrieval systems may be expected to generate healthy levels of real profit and thus achieve a greater value of goodwill.

The goodwill valuation may be defined as the capital sum which represents the capitalised value of the net profit generated, as adjusted for proprietary expenses. The 'true profit' or 'excess expected earnings' is normally monitored for the most recent three year period. Identification of trends, reconciliation of significant inconsistencies in each of the cost and expense headings as a percentage of gross income and comparison of the operational results with other similarly organised veterinary practice entities, will all influence the need to adjust the average figure. This then represents the notional anticipated annual sum.

Variances which are inevitable as part of the normal anticipated cyclical business activity will have an impact on the excess earnings level. Unexpected or non-recurring variances however, must be identified and if necessary adjusted in the calculation of adjusted net profit to arrive at the true excess expected earning for the practice.

The calculations must always be based on formal sets of accounts prepared by the practice accountants or on statutory tax and other returns appropriate for the country concerned. This will ensure that income has not been overstated and expenses have not been understated.

Management accounting information prepared by the practice owner or manager may be of assistance in examining the most recent trends in the current financial year. The objective of a detailed analysis of the accounts is to identify the financial strengths and weaknesses of the practice and to determine the excess expected earnings level which might be anticipated without regard to exceptional items.

Some expenses will need to be adjusted. For example, interest expenses which are incurred because of inadequate capitalisation is not regarded as an operating cost and is excluded. Similarly interest income resulting from a surplus of capital is also excluded.

Depreciation is similarly not a true operating cost but may be regarded as a recovery of prior capital expenditure.

Practice valuation might be described as an art as well as the result of considerable and careful examination of the financial records. The value can only ultimately be determined when the asset is sold and when the purchaser is satisfied that the price paid will reflect a fair and equitable capitalisation of the profit which he can reasonable expect will be achieved in the years following the purchase.

After making the appropriate adjustments, the expected earnings level will generally be fairly consistent as a percentage of gross. If it is not, there is usually a documented quantifiable reason for the inconsistency which must be identified.

Every practice will have a unique profit margin percentage which reflects its individual business philosophy. For this reason, attempts to base a goodwill valuation on a rule of thumb percentage of gross income are invalid since the value to the purchaser or incoming partner will depend on how much profit is retained and not on how much gross income is generated.

The basis for calculating a goodwill valuation is the net financial return which is generated to provide the potential purchaser with the means to pay back the purchase price of the practice. Any realistic valuation must respect the necessity of paying back the debt incurred in making the purchase.

The objective of the valuation method we recommend is to provide the information necessary to determine whether or not the buyer will receive a fair return on his professional time as well as on his financial investment. Ironically, the vendor will have a keen interest in the ongoing success of the practice in the purchaser's hands since, one way or another, the purchase price will be paid out of the profit which is generated.

The historical profit level must be reduced by a fair market value return for the building, land and other tangible assets, as well as for the owner's time as a veterinary clinician.

The greater the value of the practice property and other tangible assets, the greater will be the financial return which needs to be deducted from the net profit level according to the accounts and the less will be the goodwill valuation. The view could be taken that the owner's goodwill valuation is penalised for investing in an overcapitalised business that fails to generate a level of gross revenue commensurate with that investment. If profit is a measure of success, then it is important to monitor profit as a return on capital investment as well as a percentage of gross.

A successful practice requires a considerable investment of the veterinarian owner's time as a clinician in addition to his or her investment in property, vehicles, equipment and other tangible assets. An appropriate total compensation arrangement for the clinician, based upon the market conditions in the area, must be determined. The package should include a salary at least equivalent to that received by an experienced veterinarian with 5 or 6 years experience plus fringe benefits, pay-roll taxes and bonuses as appropriate.

An 80 hour work week would demand a higher salary than a 45 hour work week. The owner veterinarian with additional specialist qualifications or experience will also demand a higher total compensation package.

After deducting a fair return on capital investment and an appropriate sum in respect of the owner's investment of time as a clinician and manager, the practice valuer will determine the average net profit over a three year period and capitalise it on the basis of a realistic level of return in the order of 20% (excess expected earnings multiplied by 5).

The net profit to which we have referred above is also known as the 'excess earnings'. We think that the word 'excess' gives an erroneous impression suggesting that profit levels are ample. The contrary is often the reality. Rather, the excess expected earnings, the 'true' profit, refers to the annual anticipated earnings that become available for the practice after a fair return on investment for the tangible assets and owner veterinarian('s) time as clinician have been deducted.

Perhaps the biggest disadvantage of those methods of calculating a goodwill valuation which are based on a comparison with the total costs of the veterinarian input into the practice (employer and employee) is that they tend to confuse a very simple issue and often overstate the valuation. The practice must generate profit over and above that necessary to reward the owner as a clinician if it is to have a significant goodwill valuation.

The ultimate objective is to provide the purchasing veterinarian with the ability to make a realistic compensation package and to pay off the debt incurred in buying the practice — normally over a 10 to 15 year time span.

Before agreeing to purchase a practice, veterinarians would be strongly advise to prepare a comprehensive business plan for the immediate (two years) future of the enterprise under their management and incorporating projected income and expenditure statements and detailed cash flow forecasts.

The purchase of a partnership interest will involve additional complexities. Usually, for example, a share of the partnership assets and liabilities will need to be purchased or assumed by the incoming partner. An added complication with a partnership is that partners are jointly and separately liable for the debts of the other partners relating to the veterinary practice. Legal and accountancy advice to protect the newly acquiring partners' interests are essential.

Some Specific Issues

Valuing a Practice With Declining Profits

When a practice is declining the owner must realise that the net profit level generated over the recent years may not be deliverable in the immediate future. The purchaser then must compute the value of the practice either by reducing the capitalisation rate of recent profits or by discounting the earnings.

The views of the buyer and seller may well not coincide. The seller is unlikely to acknowledge that the practice is in decline, believes that with adequate management the practice has a rosy future but does not wish to stay committed to the business long enough to prove the point. The buyer will only buy if he or she can see an opportunity for the practice to overcome its current decline and move back into growth. Sometimes it is simply not possible to resolve the issue to the joint satisfaction of buyer and seller. In an effort to achieve a sale however, one possibility is to establish a contingent sales agreement in which the goodwill price is adjusted according to the future track record of the practice. The difficulty for the buyer is that the agreement is regarded as open-ended. The harder he works, the greater will be the profit and the more he will have to pay. Although he or she may openly express fears about the decline continuing for negotiation purposes, most buyers are optimistic about the future.

The Negotiation Process

Whilst the buyer and seller are interested in reaching an agreement, they approach the negotiation process from opposite standpoints. The buyer wants to buy at the lowest possible price. The seller wants to sell at the highest possible price. The establishment of a valuation formula is an attempt to arrive at a middle point and to determine what an independent third party might pay for the practice. The valuation formula is only a starting point for negotiation between buyer and seller. Ideally both parties will regard the independent valuation as a fair base price and then jockey for a position.

A seller may in good faith offer the buyer a fair and equitable price for the practice from the beginning. The buyer, on the other hand, may regard the proposal simply as the opening volley in the bargaining process. The negotiations may further be complicated by legal and financial advisers who may introduce esoteric issues that are seen as simply confusing the debate. Prolonged negotiation particularly if it involves considerable professional advice for both of the parties is likely to be costly and time consuming and in a number of cases the buyer and seller agree at the outset to abide by a fair and independent appraisal from a third party.

10

A Vision for the Future

It can be a dangerous and inadvisable pastime to attempt to foretell the future. We can recall many occasions over the last twenty or thirty years during which learned members of the veterinary profession have made such forecasts. Some of their prophecies have come about. Most have not. In some areas, communications and information technology for example, developments have matured faster and further than could have only been imagined a very few years ago. In others little has changed. Twenty years ago veterinarians in practice dreamed of a future in which individual practices would combine their resources and invest in expensive, high-tech central hospital premises and employ a variety of specialist expertise. It is happening, but it is very slow and patchy.

Investment in Technology

Rather than band together as the human medical profession has done, the veterinary profession has chosen to maintain the rugged, single-minded individualism that has been one of the hallmarks of the profession for decades past. Individual practices have embraced technology to the degree permitted by economics. Size has not been a significant determination of technological medical, surgical and business equipment acquisition. Rather, the willingness of the practice owner to invest in the future has been one of the most significant criteria for technological advancement.

Demographic development of the practice catchment area, competitive vendors offering similar high-tech products, the confiscatory taxing policies of government and the enthusiasm of veterinarians for their profession, have all been pivotal forces in enabling individual practices to invest in sophisticated equipment and facilities.

Generally, practices in the United States and Canada have been ready to acquire and use new technologies. Canadians and Americans, contrary to the opinions of their fellow citizens, have had one of the lowest aggregated taxing structures in the developed, modern world. Consequently, fewer man hours are required to acquire up-to-date equipment. Their professional service consuming populations have been intensely educated in the need for sophisticated medical treatment for their companion animals. Farming enterprises have likewise, discovered the wisdom of concentrating their investment in the health of the herd rather than dealing with sick individuals. With clients better educated, veterinarians have a far better opportunity to enjoy a faster and larger profit payback from their investment in technology.

The availability of equipment is also critical. When multiple vendors offer similar products, free enterprise reduces the purchase price competitively and enhances the level of service. With greater user volume, vendors have more capital to entice purchasers with more intense product promotion and advertising. Consider value added computer system vendors as an example. Suppliers are forced by the competitive demands for continued sales to provide a level of service which ensures the long term utilisation of the equipment they sell. As more veterinary customer-users experience the financial benefits of their product(s), sales of equipment, upgrades and enhancements increase.

Availability is only one factor. Affordability is another. In North America, the human medical community is obsessed with new medical equipment and gadgets. As hospital directors purchase the latest human medical technological innovations, the previously acquired equipment is discarded or sold off cheaply. The traditional beneficiary has been the veterinary medical community. Relatively up-to-date equipment, which can be used by the veterinary profession, can often be acquired at a nominal cost. In those countries where human medical consumption is not cost sensitive, the veterinary profession is provided with a greater opportunity to maintain current levels of sophistication.

The recent past will probably be replicated in the future. The dream of multiple practitioners banding together to acquire the most current technology has not generally occurred and probably will not in the future. Cherished independence will continue to transcend the logical economic arguments and individual practices which are able to do so, will continue to maintain a competitive technological edge.

The veterinary profession can be very proud of its scientific and welfare achievements. The pace of professional development continues to accelerate and it is beyond our knowledge or experience to make any attempt at looking to that scientific future. World-wide however, the profession has failed to match the pace of scientific and technical development with similar advances in understanding, researching and satisfying the needs of its clients. Similar criticism can be advanced against many of the learned professions which are service orientated. They concentrate almost exclusively on the professional needs and ambitions of their members. They neglect to give adequate consideration to the needs of their clients or potential clients, the men or women in the street, the individuals who buy or choose not to buy, the services offered.

Consumer Trends

The most important subject for a body of professionals is the profession they practice. The most important emphasis for owners or managers who are responsible for running their veterinary practice as a business, must be the market in which the practice operates. The market is always changing and we have argued the importance of taking a strategic approach to management which involves planning to deal with future events.

We would be failing in our self-imposed task if we made no mention of the future of the market in which we operate. Veterinary practice

managers would be failing to manage if they made no attempt to look into the future of their practice, their staff, their services and their market. You have to see the future to deal with the present.

None of us knows what may happen tomorrow, let alone next year or in five, ten or twenty years hence. We do believe however, that it is possible to identify consumer trends and to examine whether they have any relevance to the market for veterinary services.

Trends start small. They are not easy to spot at that stage and only the most fortunate, gifted or lucky individuals can identify a consumer trend at an early enough stage to launch a product or a service sufficiently well ahead of the competitors to make a financial fortune. By the time the direction is obvious to everybody else, the marketplace is saturated with copies or followers all trying to cash in on the trend.

By and large the challenge for the veterinary profession is not to keep ahead of the game but simply to arrive on the pitch whilst the game is still being played. Most consumer trends steadily build up to a crescendo and then plateau for some years before they decline. To some extent they are predictable. If you can identify a trend early, you can respond to the challenge and then hang on while it lasts.

Let us consider some of the trends which appear to be evident in the early 1990s and which could propel your practice through to the end of the century and beyond. Faith Popcorn has identified a number of trends which we believe could affect the marketing plan for your veterinary practice.

Trends Which May Affect Your Practice

- Cocooning; an impulse to get back home, safe and cosy when all is chaos outside (crime, AIDS, economic recession etc). Dogs, cats and other pet animals are undoubtedly perceived as characteristics of 'home' and we anticipate that the growth of dog and cat ownership is likely to continue. The growth of interest in the traditional farm animal species ie as hobby farming may also be characteristic of the 'cocooning' trend.

- Fantasy adventure; representing the need to seek relief, an escape mechanism, from stress. There are already many examples, mountain bikes, fantasy hotels, Disneyland, scuba diving, cross country walking (with a dog or dogs).
- Small indulgencies; times might be hard. Consumers may not be able to afford large expensive luxuries but they may seek little extravagancies to help them feel good. They may buy small luxuries or be prepared to pay for special, personal services from for example, their veterinary adviser. Consumers are sophisticated. They will continue to demand quality personal service at the best possible price. Value for money is all important.
- Egonomics; the 'me' decade. People don't want to be part of the mass market any more. They may appreciate the cost advantages of out of town hypermarkets and national chains but they don't want to be regarded as average. They want to be special and unique. The lesson here is to ensure that every single client is treated as a unique individual. Consumers who feel that they have special needs will seek professional advisers who are able to meet those needs and we anticipate that large animal and small animal veterinary practices will continue to be further subdivided into a wide range of practices which can offer unique specialist skills or services in a niche market.
- Cashing out; in the 1970s we worked to live. In the 1980s we lived to work. In the 1990s we simply want to live — long and well. Early retirement, a change of lifestyle, health and outdoor activities will all be perceived as increasingly valuable. It seems to us that this trend bodes well for many animal related activities.
- Down ageing; the author uses the phrase to indicate a refusal to be bound by the traditional constraints determined by age. Today's 50- and 60-year olds have more leisure, more money and want to make the best use of it all. For many life doesn't begin at 40 but at 50, 60 or 70. If you

have a significant number of retired clients you should make a special effort to cater for their special needs.
- Staying alive; the search for a happier, fitter and longer life through exercise, leisure and healthy food. The supremacy of science is being questioned. Consumers are seeking and are prepared to pay for 'natural' foods for themselves and their pets. DIY healthcare, customised diets and a growth in the development of 'foodaceuticals' reflecting a significant blurring of the edges between medicine and food. Search for and interest in 'old fashioned treatments' and alternative medicine. Much more concern with health than with illness. Perhaps the growing message from the veterinary profession will be 'how to avoid veterinary emergencies' and how to avoid medication by better management, exercise, feeding, dental care, grooming and preventive medicine.
- Consumers fighting back; As money becomes tighter consumers may be forced to buy less but buy better. They will want to buy from you, from a person and not from a system. Competition will be tough. Yesterdays standards of service are inadequate today and a recipe for failure tomorrow. The broad market will be split into niches and the niches will become smaller. The lesson for veterinary practice is that you must know who your clients are, why are they special?, what special unique services do they seek and how are you going to satisfy them?
- The need for speed; people want leisure. They want a quiet relaxed easy life. But life all around them continues to accelerate. We all tend to want to do everything. The volume of information available doubles every five years We need more time to get more done. Fast food gets faster. Consumers like to use multi-function outlets in retail parks where they can purchase carpets, furniture, DIY materials, garden equipment and so on a few short steps from the car park. There

will be considerable growth in this sort of cluster marketing and we anticipate the development of pet retail outlets 'under one roof' with veterinary hospital services, veterinary out-patient facilities, other pet animal services, recommended breeders and boarding kennels, grooming services, animal nutrition and behaviour clinics all with provision for referrals for more complex requirements and 'on line' diagnostic services by specialist veterinarians at centres of excellence in other parts of the country or even overseas.

- The decency decade; concern for the quality of the environment will increase. The professions will be taken to task if they do not put their own houses in order. The veterinary profession must take the lead in resolving the problems caused by dog fouling in urban environments.

We believe that more and more consumers will think twice or more before they make a buying decision. The rapid advances in information and communication technology will allow many more consumers to make buying decisions, place their orders and pay their bills at home. They may be prepared to go shopping if parking is easy, if it is all 'under one roof' and if the excursion can be perceived as a pleasant outing perhaps with an element of theatre as well as shopping. We think however that one of the veterinary marketing niches which will need to be satisfied will be a modern, high-tech and sophisticated home visiting clinical service.

Veterinary practices which have not invested in computer technology will become very much the exception. We are sure that the computer client and patient database will be perceived as one of the most valuable practice assets and that it will be used in conjunction with mailmerge and other techniques as a powerful, effective and economical marketing tool to enable the practice to conduct regular in-depth marketing studies amongst their existing clients and to target a range of service and market initiatives.

We hope that this book will contribute to an understanding of the relationship between professional excellence and fair profit. We have endeavoured to promote the importance of veterinary practice as a business as well as a profession. We trust that an awareness of the interdependence of the traditional art and science of veterinary practice with the economic necessity of financial success is promoted by our thoughts, opinions and commentary through this book.

The Challenge Ahead

The challenge then for the practising arm of the veterinary profession in the 1990s and beyond will be to commit increasing resources to scientific and clinical continuing education for professional and support staff and at the same time to involve them all in business management issues.

If the right balance is struck between management and clinical matters and if practice owners, leaders and employees are satisfied with nothing less than total quality in everything they do, the practising arm of the veterinary profession can face the future with confidence.

APPENDIX

A Business Plan for your Practice

The final section of this book is concerned with the task of preparing a business plan for your own veterinary practice.

You are about to develop a strategic plan for the practice for the next two years and then convert that broad strategy into detailed plans for action.

Before you start, remember why you need a plan and what specific steps you have to take:

1. Why Plan?

- to reach a defined destination — where are you going?
- to avoid failure.
- to ensure that everyone in the practice is working to the same objective.
- to set targets, to monitor and measure achievement.

2. Mission Statement — Do you need one? why?

- to identify a common understanding amongst the partners.
- to provide a message to your employees.
- as a message to external stakeholders, clients and investors.

3. Your Present Strategy

- what is it?
- how did it develop?
- what has changed?
    external
    internal

4. Formulating a New Strategy

- what needs changing
- S.W.O.T. analysis
- stakeholders expectations
- broad objectives

5. External Influences

- economic
- ecological
- technical
- social
- legal
- political
- other

6. Role of the Leader — You and your colleagues.

- What is your VISION?
- What makes your practice special?
  - market segment, image, style, the perception of the practice by staff and clients, performance expectations, distinctive features.

7. Objectives — be explicit

- who will be required to set and implement them?
- what about profits?
- what about market share?
- what about growth?
- what about your employees?
- what about your services?
- what social objectives?
- consider the time scale
- consider priorities within objectives

8. Managing Change

The '7-S model' demonstrates that successful change depends on:

- shared values (does everyone in the team understand the mission and goals of the practice? Are they strongly supported and is the team cohesive and working in the same direction?)
- staff
- style
- structure
- strategy
- skills
- system

9. A Strategic Plan — is not merely an extended budget but involves ideas as well as numbers.

- objectives
- S.W.O.T. analysis
- analysis of the market
- analysis of competitors
- strategic options
- strategic choices
- resource needs
- plan
    organise
    control
- people plans

10. Serving the Client — what do they want? (ask the front line staff)

- talk to clients
- capture the information (reception desk surveys)
- talk to the front line staff — often
- identify the inhibitors to service
- remove the inhibitors (maybe the 'system' or even partners inhibit the services your clients want)

11. Staff — Do you have the right number of people with the appropriate skills in their correct roles?

Consider:
- what skills are required?
- do you have them?
- are they changing?
- can you or your staff develop new skills? how?
- create a learning environment
- create enthusiasm for learning
- develop innovative ability
- invest in the learning process

12. Now Some 'Don'ts — Whatever the strategic process Don't:

- choke the system with irrelevant data
- produce plans which no one believes in
- produce plans for other people to implement
- believe in your forecasts entirely.

Your business plan must BELONG to the whole practice

THE PLAN — Remember THE PLAN must be realistic, clear, easy to follow, and sufficiently detailed for you to use as a blueprint. Your plan is custom built for your practice and written by the users who are committed to it. The objective is to produce a 'route map' for the practice for two years.

SOME TIPS

Avoid shortcuts. It will be very tempting to avoid the first sections — the analysis of your practice history and the current situation. It is very important that you complete each stage to help you decide your objectives from now on.

- Keep your comments clear and concise.
- Double check all documentation that involves numbers. Make sure that all your percentages add up to 100.
- Maintain a personal practice library of documents and information which will assist you to develop future business plans.

- The success of your plan will depend on the support of your colleagues and staff. Take every opportunity of involving them in the planning process. Be clear at the outset that your success will be their success and that everyone involved will benefit. You must take the lead but don't try to do the whole thing on your own. It is no good drafting a plan in isolation and then expecting everybody involved to carry it out. Involve everybody in deciding where you are now, where you are going and how you are going to get there.
- Review the completed plan with your staff and colleagues, modify and refine it until you are satisfied. Once it is complete refer to it frequently.
- Seek help and advice and the appropriate expertise. Remember that you must write the plan. The greatest value of the exercise is the time and thought that you and your colleagues put into it.
- Write down everything that is relevant but do not let the planning process be an excuse for failing to do what you know needs doing now.
- At an appropriate stage, talk your plan through with your bank manager and accountant, and keep them informed as matters proceed.

GET STARTED

Finally remember that the first step is often the most difficult. GET STARTED NOW OR YOU MAY NEVER GET STARTED AT ALL:

IF YOU FAIL TO PLAN YOU MAY WELL BE PLANNING TO FAIL.

Index